THE
CANCER PATIENT'S
HANDBOOK

Also by Mary-Ellen Siegel

Her Way

Chemotherapy: Your Weapon Against Cancer
    (co-author: Ezra M. Greenspan, M.D.)

What Every Man Should Know About His Prostate
    (co-author: Monroe E. Greenberger, M.D.)

More Than a Friend: Dogs with a Purpose
    (co-author: Hermine M. Koplin)

Reversing Hair Loss

THE CANCER PATIENT'S HANDBOOK

Everything You Need to Know About Today's Care and Treatment

Mary-Ellen Siegel, M.S.W.

Senior Teaching Associate
Department of Community Medicine (Social Work)
Mount Sinai School of Medicine
City University of New York

Foreword by
Ezra M. Greenspan, M.D.

Clinical Professor of Medicine
Associate Chief, Division of Oncology
Mount Sinai School of Medicine
City University of New York

Walker and Company ☀ **New York**

First published in the United States of America
in 1986 by the Walker Publishing Company, Inc.

Published simultaneously in Canada by John Wiley & Sons
Canada, Limited, Rexdale, Ontario.

Library of Congress Cataloging-in-Publication Data

Siegel, Mary-Ellen.
    The cancer patient's handbook.

    Bibliography: p.
    Includes index.
    1. Cancer—Popular works. I. Title. [DNLM:
1. Neoplasms—therapy—popular works. QZ 201 S571c]
RC263.S487   1986   616.99′4   86-13247
ISBN 0-8027-0898-6
ISBN 0-8027-7290-0 (pbk.)

Printed in the United States of America

10   9   8   7   6   5   4   3   2

Contents

To Hermine,
who always kept her promise.

Author's Note

For the sake of literary uniformity, the patient is referred to as *you*, and the physician is frequently referred to as *he*. I am fully aware that women are represented in every medical specialty and that many readers are being treated by highly qualified family physicians, surgeons, radiotherapists, and oncologists who are women.

Foreword

We live in an age of medical miracles so commonplace that they are taken for granted by all of us. Since 1940, the magic of chemotherapy with antibiotics and synthetic chemicals has prevented millions of deaths from pneumonia, mastoiditis, scarlet fever, syphilis, typhoid, lung abscess and many other infections. Tuberculosis, the killer of millions worldwide, came under control with three-drug combination chemotherapy. Thus, life expectancy has suddenly and markedly increased in recent decades. With this progress, cancer, the scourge of millions, has come to affect one out of three American families.

At the same time, improvement in surgical techniques, anesthesia and intravenous patient support has made major surgery safer than ever before. Advances in X-ray therapy have broadened the potential of treating cancers confined to a single location in the body. It is now estimated that 50 percent of patients with various kinds of local cancers can look forward to virtual cure with surgery and/or radiotherapy.

Yet every year 350,000 Americans die from cancer that surgery or radiotherapy alone could not cure, while more than a million are living with cancer that has spread to other parts of the body. The hope of this million is that systemic changes in the body induced by drugs, hormones, and other agents will cure them or prolong their survival by halting the disseminated tumors.

Since 1960, dramatic clinical benefits have been achieved in an increasing number of different kinds of difficult cancers. In the curative category are acute lymphatic leukemia, lymphomas, Hodgkin's disease, testicular cancer and osteosarcomas. Long-term control and cure can now be expected in a significant number of patients with breast cancer and, to a lesser extent, in ovarian cancer. Important increases in survival are now being made in a variety of other cancers, including small-cell cancer of the lung, bladder cancer, prostate cancer, and others. Despite this remarkable progress, the patient with disseminated cancer feels beleaguered and under constant life threat. Conflicting medical advice from physicians, relatives, friends, and the media, and the uncertainty of one's future, combine to create confusion, anxiety and even despair.

When the physician initially suspects that a patient might have cancer he or she may order a number of complex and sophisticated tests; if the suspicion is confirmed the physician will then order tests to determine the extent of the disease. This process can leave a patient in a state of anxious suspense. When diagnosis is complete, and treatment is to begin, the patient often worries: Am I getting the best treatment available today?

It is the purpose of this book to dispel some of this cloud by providing vital information on so many of the problems and questions facing patients, family, friends, and health professionals.

The role of the medical oncologist is particularly paramount in cancer management because this is the physician responsible for the total care of the patient. Communication and understanding between them is an essential key to living with cancer. Indeed, the psychological attitudes and adjustments of patients may play a significant role in how patients cope with the diverse methods of therapy employed today.

THE CANCER PATIENT'S HANDBOOK acts as a guide to the seemingly innumerable questions and problems of patients with cancer and to their ever changing medical status. Most patients wish to know the facts surrounding the medical management of their cancer. Despite the best of intentions, physicians are often too busy to assume fully the role of patient-educator. This book serves as a constant supplement and interpreter of important information, and together with the physician, and other health professionals such as nurses, social workers, counselors, and psychologists, is a reassuring presence. It is an important aide in communication between doctor, patient, and family, and strengthens the essential bond between them.

Ezra M. Greenspan, M.D.

Clinical Professor of Medicine (Oncology)
Mount Sinai School of Medicine
City University of New York
New York

Medical Director
The Chemotherapy Foundation, Inc.

Acknowledgments

The following people have given freely of their time and expertise preceding and during the period I was writing this book. In addition, many of them kindly read portions or all of the manuscript and made valuable suggestions. Others have taught me much that helped me in my own work with patients, and I am most grateful to all of them.

They include Claire Bennett, M.S.W.; Arlene Berger, M.S.W.; Sally Bishop, R.N.; Luanne Brogna, R.N.; Kay Coltoff, M.S.W.; Jack Dalton, M.D.; Eugene Friedman, M.D.; Allen Gribetz, M.D.; Michael Gribetz, M.D.; Barbara Keyes, R.N.; Eva Levine, R.N.; Louis Lapid, M.D.; James McVey, R.R.T.; Phyllis Mervis, M.S.W.; Daniel Present, M.D.; Helen Rehr, D.S.W.; Gary Rosenberg, Ph.D; Jack Rudick, M.D.; Penny Schwartz, M.S.W.; Sidney Silverstone, M.D.; Samuel Waxman, M.D.; Cecilia Wilfinger, R.N.; and Elizabeth DeVito, M.L.S., and others of the Levy Library staff—all of the Mount Sinai School of Medicine in New York; Michael Feinstein, M.D., of North Shore Hospital and Long Island Jewish Medical Center in New York; Jimmie Holland, M.D., of Memorial Sloan-Kettering Medical Center in New York; Joel Kassimir, M.D., of New York University Medical Center; Shirley Cox of the Chemotherapy Foundation, Inc.; Jan AufderHeide of Upjohn; Carolyn Messner, M.S.W., of Cancer Care, Inc.; Sirini Stockwell of the American Cancer Society; Linda Anderson of the National Cancer Institute; Ellyn Bushkin, R.N., oncology nurse clinician; Judith Nierenberg, R.N., director of educational resources for the American Journal of Nursing Company; Austin Kutscher, D.D.S.; Marcia G. Fishman, R.N. and Brian Morgan, Ph.D., of the Columbia Presbyterian Medical Center; and the entire staff of the Hillcrest Branch of the Queensborough Public Library System.

My family, nuclear and extended, as always, encourage and sustain me. Many of them know too well what it is like to live through cancer.

Richard Winslow's encouragement, patience, suggestions, and assistance are enormously appreciated.

Helpful beyond all expectations were Daniel Martin, M.D., of Memorial Sloan-Kettering Hospital and the Catholic Medical Center;

Lynn Ratner, M.D., of the Mount Sinai School of Medicine and Lenox Hill Hospital; Robert Frank, R.Ph.; Larry Norton, M.D.; and Jaclyn Silverman of the Mount Sinai School of Medicine.

Many of the concepts and portions of the chapter on pain were derived from material prepared and written by Robert Frank, R.Ph., with his permission.

I am particularly grateful to Ezra M. Greenspan, M.D., clinical professor of medicine (oncology), of the Mount Sinai School of Medicine. With kindness and brilliance, he has cared for members of my family; he has also encouraged and informed me in my own work with and for cancer patients. As medical director of the Chemotherapy Foundation, Inc., he has made research and information available to the medical and health-care professions and to the public alike, helping countless cancer patients receive the best treatment possible. Without him this book would not have come to fruition.

Note: A portion of all royalties from this book will be donated to the Chemotherapy Foundation, Inc., 183 Madison Avenue, New York, NY 10016.

Introduction

Cancer. There was a time, not so long ago, when the word wasn't even whispered. Occasionally, words were substituted. "Chronic blood disease," "women's trouble," "prostate condition," "asthma," "emphysema," and even "arthritis" were used to describe the disease that everyone thought was a death warrant.

Now we often hear murmurings of "neoplasms," "malignancy," and "tumors." These words don't have the same harshness as cancer and it is easier to pretend that a life-threatening illness doesn't exist.

Increasingly, people speak more openly of cancer. Most patients want to know, and are told by their doctors, if they have cancer. Families no longer keep it a secret from the patient and from others. Since the mid-1970s there have been many changes in the public's attitudes toward cancer. This is due to the medical strides made in controlling and curing cancer and to reports of these advances by responsible medical journalists. Also, people today show willingness to be more open about many personal and private matters in general. Everyone knows some people who are cured or show no evidence of having had cancer.

But still, when people learn they have cancer, often they cannot face it. They feel as if they are having a nightmare from which they will awaken, or that the phone will ring and a voice will say, "We have discovered that we made a mistake. You don't have cancer at all." It's quite normal to have these feelings of denial.

Every day we read or hear about ordinary people who have become extraordinary at coping with cancer and comparable adversities. These stories are inspiring, and sometimes we can adopt some of the characteristics or behavior of these "quiet heroes." But sometimes we can't.

Most of us confront everyday setbacks without any reordering of priorities, change in life-style, or rebirth of religion. We proceed through life with a hopeful attitude: working, living, loving, and enjoying good times throughout our decades on earth. When cancer strikes, we experience it as a serious crisis, but not an absolute disaster. The experience of coping with cancer can sometimes make us stronger, sometimes more fragile, and sometimes only slightly changed.

As soon as your family physician suspects you have cancer, it is important to get a complete diagnosis and to begin treatment. *Early treatment, like early diagnosis, ensures the best chance for cure or long-time survival.*

Before beginning any kind of treatment (surgery, radiation, or chemotherapy) you should seek a second opinion regarding your diagnosis and planned treatment. The American Medical Association recommends (except in the case of emergency surgery) that people get a second opinion before agreeing to *any* surgical procedure. Many medical experts advise that you should also get an opinion from a medical oncologist (a cancer specialist) to learn if he agrees with the diagnosis and if surgery or another treatment is indicated.

At one time surgery was the only effective treatment for cancer. Today, in many instances, surgery is not recommended. This does not mean the cancer is inoperable (usually interpreted by patients and family as "too far gone") but that other methods of treatment may be more effective, or that surgery may be planned *following* other treatments.

In the pages that follow, I will answer the questions that patients and their families most frequently ask. Cancer patients (and those who care for or about them) need to live as normal a life as possible while going through months or years of treatment. In these pages you will learn how to go about finding the information you want, and how to shut off what you really *don't* want or need to know.

This book will tell you most of what you want to know, but you may also consider reading in greater detail about your particular kind of cancer. The appendix "For Further Reading" lists several titles. Your librarian can help you seek out magazines and medical journals with relevant information, and the counselors at the Cancer Information Service (see Appendix VI for telephone numbers) may be able to guide you in seeking additional information.

This book is a guide through the maze of treatments and health-care services that are available. It will tell you if treatment is standard, experimental, unproven, or even disproved.

It will discuss learning to live with and through cancer, adapting to it so that it does not completely take over your life. Cancer may not make you a hero, nor will it guarantee you hidden strengths to make you a poet, a saint, a better parent, a more loving spouse, or a pillar of society. But this book will guide you, the patient, in your travels through the rough times. Like a guidebook to a foreign country, it will discuss the basics of making known your needs and desires to your family, friends, coworkers, physicians, and other health-care professionals. Most important, it will show you how you can work together with all these people to make your treatment as effective as possible.

Some people say the side effects of the treatment are the worst part of the entire cancer experience, but you will learn how to better tolerate and even minimize them. I will talk about the foods to eat and to avoid. I will also show you how to keep careful, important records.

This book will *not* dwell on *why* or *how* you got cancer, but it *will* teach you survival tactics that can increase your life span, make you feel in control, and help you see yourself as a hopeful survivor.

Section One

FINDING OUT ABOUT CANCER

Chapter 1
What Is Cancer?

Cancer is a general term used to describe the groups of diseases characterized by abnormal cell growth in the body. Cancer cells do not usually stay in any one place; instead, they move around, crowding between normal cells and even penetrating them. Unchecked by medical intervention, these cells tend to spread to distant body sites.

Different and continually improving modes of treatment—the major ones are surgery, chemotherapy, and radiotherapy—are proving successful in combating cancer. Occasionally, cancer seems to disappear without treatment in what is called a spontaneous remission. This occurs because, in some way that is not yet understood, the body's own immune system has been mobilized to virtually destroy or even "evict" the cancer from the body.

The human body is made up of cells, all of which have specific purposes. These cells continually grow and divide in order to replace those cells that have died or become worn out. Blood cells and skin cells are examples of cells that are constantly being replaced. Normal cells seem to "know" when to stop growing and dividing. Normal division is more rapid in infancy and childhood (to allow for growth of the individual) than in adulthood, when cell reproduction occurs only to maintain life. For example, wounds heal, but the cells reproduce only enough to replace the damage, and then cease to grow. Other cells, such as those of hair and fingernails, may grow continually, but they do not spread to other parts of the body.

Cancer cells differ from normal cells in many ways. They have an irregular, disordered appearance when viewed under a microscope. Unlike normal cells, cancer cells serve no useful function, nor do they wear out and die like normal cells. Instead, these malignant cells continue to divide and multiply, reproducing themselves, invading and destroying surrounding tissues. In so doing, they deprive the normal cells of nourishment, which can cause weight loss and create obstructions to normal body functioning.

1

Tumors

A tumor is a purposeless swelling or enlargement in the body. A tumor can be either benign (noncancerous) or malignant (made up of a mass of cancer cells). When the mass of cells remains in the site where they originated, the tumor is said to be *localized*. Cells that have spread to another part of the body but are confined to a specific area are described as *regional*. Cells that have spread, or *metastasized*, throughout the body by way of the blood or lymph system can create new tumors.

Cancer cells can spread slowly or rapidly, in an orderly or chaotic fashion. Cancer that begins in one part of the body may show up somewhere else weeks, months, or years later. Scientists and individual physicians cannot always predict the course of any specific cancer.

Although cancer cells frequently form tumors, it is important to remember that not every tumor is composed of cancerous cells.

When a tumor or growth is removed from a patient, it is examined by a pathologist, a physician who is especially trained to study and evaluate the characteristics, causes, and effects of disease by use of laboratory tests and other methods. The pathologist determines if the tumor is benign or malignant.

A benign tumor can be very small or can grow huge, interfering with or obstructing neighboring tissues or organs. Cells from a benign tumor do not spread to other parts of the body.

Cells from a malignant tumor, on the other hand, may have already traveled to other parts of the body (metastasized) *before* the surgeon removes it. Despite the surgeon's assurance that "we got it all out," patients with malignancies should continue to have frequent and regular checkups after surgery.

Types of Cancer

To appreciate the difficulty in fully understanding cancer, one must realize that cancer is not just one disease but many related diseases. It can arise in any organ or tissue of the body. Many categories of cancer have been identified, and within these categories there are many variations. A particular form of cancer is generally described by its location in the body and by the type of cells of which it is composed. Carcinomas, sarcomas, lymphomas, leukemias, and myelomas are just a few of these cell types.

Carcinomas are cancers that grow in tissues that cover or line the body or internal organs. Lungs, breasts, colon, intestines, and skin are common sites of origin for carcinomas.

Sarcomas originate in bones and in tissues that connect or lie between organs and skin, and they may spread throughout the blood or lymphatic system. An example is osteogenic sarcoma, which develops in bone-forming cells.

Lymphomas form in the lymphatic system, most commonly the lymph nodes. The lymphatic system is a complex network of channels and ducts throughout the body that transports lymph, a clear fluid which bathes the tissues and is discharged into the bloodstream by way of the thoracic duct. The lymph nodes are small oval structures that act as sieves, filtering lymph and fighting infection. Lymphomas can also arise in the spleen and lymph glands. Hodgkin's disease is an example of a lymphoma.

Leukemias are cancers of the blood or circulatory system, and usually arise in the bone marrow, where blood cells are produced.

Myelomas are those cancers that form tumors composed of cells normally found in bone marrow. Myeloma may form simultaneously in many sites, most frequently in ribs, vertebrae, and pelvic bones. Examples are multiple myeloma and osteogenic myeloma.

A more detailed description of specific cancers will be found in Chapter 9.

Because there are so many varieties of cancer, there is a wide range of treatments and treatment plans. When planning treatment, doctors take many factors into consideration, including the extent of the disease and the general condition of the patient. Cancer is treatable, but not always predictable, so responses to surgery, radiation, and chemotherapy vary from one patient to another. Different patients with the same diagnosis may react quite differently to one treatment. Even within the same individual, major changes in the nature of the cancer can occur, so a patient who has not been responding well to a particular treatment may suddenly begin to make a remarkable recovery if the doctor persists with that treatment; or another therapy altogether may prove effective. Every case is unique.

What Causes Cancer?

Among the most common external factors that can contribute to the development of cancer are smoking; excessive alcohol consumption; continued exposure to sunlight, radiation, or certain chemicals found in the environment; and diets high in fat and low in fiber. Smoking and lung cancer are closely related. Heavy drinkers have a much greater chance of developing cancer of the mouth, throat, and esophagus. But nonsmokers may also develop lung cancer, and nondrinkers may of course develop head and neck cancers. And everyone knows a three-pack-a-day smoker who lived to a ripe old age and died of unrelated causes.

Most studies today indicate that carcinogens (substances known to cause cancer in either laboratory animals or humans), like those mentioned above, *plus* other factors (including hereditary predispositions) must be present before any given individual develops cancer. In some instances, viruses have been shown to be influential in the development of cancer. People can reduce many of the risks of developing cancer but can do little about hereditary factors. Nor can they do anything about carcinogens they may have been exposed to many years ago, in childhood or even before birth.

We all have a natural immune system that protects us from a host of illnesses and diseases, and which can help us recover from some that do develop. Many scientists today believe that some cancers may result in part from a breakdown in this immune system, but no specific types of cancer have yet been clearly or exclusively implicated. What makes this system break down? Many studies suggest that stress and heredity could do damage, but so far no one has proved that this is a crucial factor. Some speculate that a lack of exposure to numerous infections, protection with antibiotics and modern sanitation may also lower the immune system.

Recent research indicates that certain genes (the basic hereditary messages carried in the form of DNA) may be "turned on" to trigger the development of malignant cells. These particular genes are called oncogenes, or cancer genes, and are thought to interact with carcinogens to cause specific cancers. As yet, the "switch" that "turns on" these genes has not been identified.

Many causes of cancer are known; some are still completely unknown. Cancer is *not* contagious; bruises do not develop into cancer, although these myths persist.

Pages and pages could be devoted to the causes of cancer; indeed, there are books that devote themselves strictly to ways of warding off cancer. People can and should exert control over their life-style and diet, but they cannot always avoid environmental factors, nor can they dictate their heredity.

Most important, one *cannot* turn back the clock. If you already have developed cancer, there is little to be gained by focusing or dwelling upon how this occurred. Most cancers cannot be ascribed to any single specific cause, although it's only human to try to find a reason for everything. Thus, many people have the idea, buried deep inside, that illnesses are caused by their own thoughts or behavior or that

someone or something has somehow caused this. They may feel helpless because of heredity or some other factor beyond their control. And
so when they develop cancer, they tend to look for someone or something to blame.

Self-reproach and blame may resurface many times during the
course of your illness. "Why did I wait so long to go to the doctor?"
and "I've done everything the doctors told me to do, so why aren't I
better yet?"

Although these feelings, concerns, and questions are natural, there
are other, far more important matters that the newly diagnosed cancer
patient needs to focus on. When all is said and done, the best way to
start learning to live through cancer and to fight it is to find the best
treatment available. And you *can* get excellent treatment almost anywhere in the United States or Canada today. As soon as cancer is either
suspected or diagnosed, embarking on that treatment should be your
first priority.

Is It Really Cancer?

No doubt you are aware of the seven warning signs of cancer,
which the American Cancer Society displays in many public places:

Change in bowel or bladder habits.
A sore that does not heal.
Unusual bleeding or discharge.
Thickening or lump in the breast or elsewhere.
Indigestion or difficulty in swallowing.
Obvious change in a wart or mole.
Nagging cough or hoarseness.

In addition to these warning signs, you should trust your own feelings about your body. Extreme tiredness, weakness, dizziness, sharp or
dull chronic pain, sudden or constant unaccountable weight loss or
gain, swelling in any part of your body, and personality changes should
all be reported to your doctor.

Your family doctor, or the health center or clinic in your neighborhood, should take any of your complaints seriously. Any of the above
may be symptoms of something that will go away by itself or with minor
treatment. But that is no reason to ignore symptoms. And just as you
should trust your feelings when your body is telling you "something is
wrong," so you should trust your instincts if you feel your doctor is not
taking your symptoms seriously or is urging you to wait too long before
further investigation.

Even if your doctor suspects cancer, there is seldom an emergency.
A few days or a week or two, unless you are already seriously ill, will

probably not be crucial. On the basis of his examination and some basic blood tests, X rays, or cytology tests (analysis of tissue), your family doctor may suspect or confirm that cancer is present.

At this time you should see a cancer specialist (an oncologist) before proceeding with further tests or treatment, to be certain that you are getting the best possible care from the outset.

Chapter 2
Getting the Best Care

Your family doctor will probably be able to recommend a physician or clinic that specializes in cancer. Be sure that the doctor to whom you have been referred is *a properly trained specialist* in treating cancer patients. It may take some phoning and investigating to find such a cancer specialist, but no matter where you live, you can receive the finest "state of the art" care for cancer.

Cancer is such an unpredictable disease, both in its natural course and in its treatment, that only highly skilled planning with individual attention by specialists can assure you the best possible care.

Medical oncologists are physicians who have been fully trained in both internal medicine as well as the management and supervision of cancer treatment. They have had advanced training in a hospital approved by the American Board of Internal Medicine and have passed the certifying examination. Many are also board-certified in oncology, but as this subspecialty was not formally recognized until 1972, there are some very fine cancer specialists who do not have certification, merely because their training dates back to the 1950s or 1960s. It is worth noting that some internists who have been treating cancer patients for many years, have kept abreast of all the latest findings, and have had some formal training in oncology may be able to provide you with good care.

Medical oncologists are sometimes referred to as **chemotherapists,** because they assume the responsibility of treating cancer with drugs (chemotherapy).

Surgical oncologists are surgeons who are board-certified in surgery and have chosen to specialize in surgical care of cancer patients. There is no board certification in surgical oncology, but many surgeons who specialize in cancer surgery have been trained in a cancer hospital and are members of the Society of Surgical Oncology, Society of Gynecologic Oncologists, or the Society of Head and Neck Surgeons. There is a small group of physicians who are board-certified in the specialty of gynecological oncology.

Radiotherapists, often called radiation oncologists or radiation thera-pists, are physicians whose specialty is treating cancer patients using various forms of radiation. They have received lengthy, formal training in evaluating and treating cancer patients with all forms of radiation. They are board-certified in radiology, with a special certificate in thera-peutic radiology. Patients are referred to radiotherapists by their medi-cal oncologists or surgeons.

Some or all of these specialists, along with the cancer patient's primary physician, may form the team that will care for the cancer patient. Many experts believe that even if your family physician has experience treating cancer, you should at least *consult* with a medical oncologist once cancer has been suspected or diagnosed. During this initial consultation, the medical oncologist will verify precise diagnosis, help to establish the best method of treating you, and then continue to monitor your progress. The medical oncologist's training and experi-ence enable him to observe, recognize, and often predict whether your cancer is spreading, shrinking, or lying dormant. He will refer you to other specialists and work closely with them whenever necessary. Some people feel that whenever possible, a medical oncologist should be the cancer patient's *primary* physician, the doctor to whom the patient turns with *all* medical concerns, because he is the one best able to evaluate if any of those problems are related to the cancer.

There are some specialists who are highly qualified to treat partic-ular kinds of cancer even if their chief specialty is not cancer itself. Some gynecologists who are not board-certified in gynecological on-cology can still competently treat women with cancer of the reproduc-tive organs. Some urologists have also made a specialty of treating men with prostatic, testicular, and other urological cancers. Pulmonary spe-cialists and thoracic surgeons may be very experienced in treating pa-tients with lung cancer. Hematologists, whose specialty is diseases of the blood and blood-making tissues, often treat cancer patients, espe-cially those with lymphomas or leukemias. Gastroenterologists treat many cancers of the digestive tract.

In many locations, particularly in large medical centers that treat numerous cancer patients, it is entirely possible to obtain the most modern and effective treatment for your cancer from one of these spe-cialists. In smaller communities, a gynecologist or gastroenterologist may not have the opportunity to treat large numbers of cancer patients and hence lacks adequate experience to do the work of an oncologist. But wherever you live, you should definitely consider having a consul-tation with a cancer specialist.

HOW TO FIND A MEDICAL ONCOLOGIST

It is not always practical to have a medical oncologist as your primary physician if none practices near your home. But even if you live too far away for regular visits, you can still have the full benefits of an oncologist's training and expertise. Your family doctor can arrange a consultation with one, or with the oncology department of the nearest medical center. Even if *you* don't go there, your family doctor can send reports to, and have a full discussion with, such a specialist. You can then be sure you are getting the latest available treatment. If you require drugs, your family doctor can obtain these drugs and administer them to you. You both can continue to consult frequently and regularly with the oncologist via visits and reports (written or by telephone).

There is no need to be embarrassed to ask your family doctor for this consultation. The physician who has your best interests at heart will be eager to work with you in your fight against cancer. It is impossible for any doctor to be the complete expert in all aspects of health care. One of the hallmarks of a good family physician is knowing when to seek consultations, and to refer a patient elsewhere when appropriate. A diagnosis of cancer is certainly one of those times.

If your family doctor cannot recommend an oncologist, or says he doesn't perceive the need for the referral, do *not* accept this statement passively. You can phone the nearest major teaching hospital (one that is connected with a medical school, if possible) and ask for the department or division of oncology. Ask this department to suggest appropriate specialists from their staff. Your local medical society (call your local Department of Health if you can't find the phone number) may also be able to make suggestions. You can also write or phone the American Society of Clinical Oncology (see Appendix VI) for names of members near you. All members are board-certified or board-eligible in oncology (that is, they have already passed the specialty examinations or their training has made them eligible to take the exams), and one of them is likely to be near enough for you to consult.

The reference librarian at your local library can also help you find the *Directory of Medical Specialists*, where you can check credentials of any physician who is recommended to you. This source may also be useful in your search for a cancer specialist, since they are cross-indexed by geographical location.

The National Cancer Institute of the U.S. Department of Health and Human Services has designated twenty-one comprehensive cancer centers located at major teaching hospitals throughout the United States. Their central office of Cancer Communications can refer you to the one nearest you, but they will usually not give you the names of individual oncologists who can offer you direct, continuing medical care. These comprehensive centers offer excellent care, and if your cancer is an unusual one, such a center may be the best place for treatment. You can also use this center as a starting point from which to get referrals for individual physicians, if that is your preference.

To reach the nationwide Cancer Information Service (CIS) from most areas, call 1-800-4-CANCER during business hours and you will automatically be connected to their office in your own area. See Appendix VI for complete details. These offices, each associated with a major medical center, are staffed by people who are prepared to explain medical terms, advise on local treatment facilities and resources, and provide facts about specific types of cancer.

Be thorough, but don't waste precious time with an unnecessarily long search for medical care.

When you feel confident that the specialist you have been referred to has the necessary credentials and experience to supervise or give you direct care, you should think about other aspects of your forthcoming relationship with this physician.

Does the doctor have a close associate who will be familiar with me in the event that my own doctor is on vacation or unavailable when I need him? All doctors have someone who "covers" for them when they are unavailable, but the covering physician may not be completely familiar with you personally. If that is important to you, then be sure to choose an oncologist who has a regular covering physician, an office partner or an associate. Plan to meet this doctor *prior* to need.

Will the oncologist remain in contact with my family physician, so that they can continue to cooperate in my care? If you are eager to continue your relationship with your family physician (perhaps this doctor has known you for many years, treats other members of the family, and is geographically or emotionally close to you), it is important that the oncologist understand and agree to such contact.

If the oncologist is going to become my primary physician, will I be able to get to the office on a regular basis, or whenever I feel the need? If the oncologist's office is far away or otherwise difficult to get to, this may be a difficult situation. Is there someone who can take you there if you are sometimes unable to travel alone? If geographic location looms as a problem, it is important that the oncologist be willing to cooperate with your local family doctor.

Do I have a good rapport with this oncologist—and do I really like him? Ideally, you should be able to answer yes to this question. But perhaps the oncologist you've chosen seems cold, distant, or not as open as you would like. If you live in a large city, or there is more than one qualified oncologist near you, *find another doctor.* But if there really is no choice (and this may be the case in some locations), my advice is to decide whether you would rather have a warm, caring physician who isn't really an expert on cancer *or* an impersonal physician whose expertise and experience does lie in the area of cancer.

I know where my choice would lie: with the experienced cancer expert. And by the time you finish reading this book, you may learn ways to make such an expert more responsive to your needs.

In the past, you probably chose physicians who were well trained, but you didn't insist they be among the world's leading experts in their specialties. In all likelihood, you also developed good rapport with them.

Cancer is another matter. You are dealing with a life-threatening illness, one in which chances for control and cure are increasing year by year. Cure rates are highest where the patient is treated in the most skilled way possible. You need and deserve the best in medical care for cancer. Don't settle for less.

Chapter 3
Diagnosis and Staging

The evaluation process by which the type or extent of cancer is determined is important for planning treatment. There is no single test that can yield all this information, so instead, a combination of tests and procedures is necessary to establish a complete diagnosis. A complete diagnosis includes information about the precise type of cancer, where it has originated and whether or not is has penetrated or spread throughout your body, and whether it is dependent on various hormones for growth. These factors will contribute to the formulation of a treatment plan. When you have chosen the doctor or clinic where you will be treated, this diagnostic evaluation, called a *workup* or *staging*, will begin.

Most medical centers and cancer specialists have agreed upon definite stages by which to describe the state of a patient's cancer. Stage I usually means that the cancer is limited to the organ or area where it began. Stages II, III, and IV involve further development of the cancer. Within each stage, there are still further classifications.

In many types of cancer, stage I is easily cured. But in others, this same stage may be difficult and complicated to treat. Likewise, Stage IV in some types of cancer is highly treatable. But in other cancers it may require very intensive treatment to effect remission or cure.

Today, most cancers are treatable, and many are curable. I cannot say it often enough: *Cancers differ widely from one another, and so do individual responses to treatment.*

People's responses to learning that they have cancer also vary. And people have different ways of wanting to hear the news. Some would like to be told by their doctor when they are alone with him; others would prefer to be told in the presence of a loved one. Still others would prefer to learn about it after their family has been told. Few people want to learn it over the phone. It would be wise to discuss this with your physician before your tests are complete—so that you can hear the results in a way that is most comfortable for you.

But still, no matter how you learn that you have cancer, the news will be difficult to cope with. In Chapter 16 I will discuss some of the ways in which people are emotionally affected by cancer in themselves or family members.

When you learn you have cancer, you may just sit down and cry. Or you may deny the news, pushing the diagnosis out of your mind. You may even wonder aloud why your doctor hasn't told you anything when indeed you have been told a great deal. You may become so overwhelmed with the diagnosis that you can think of little else, and become very depressed or angry. Family members may react similarly—or they may become overprotective and try to take over your life, making you feel as if you no longer have control over anything. Occasionally, family members are so overwhelmed with fear, anger, or resentment that they retreat from their usual relations with you. Or to ward off their own feelings of sorrow, pity, guilt, or some other uncomfortable feeling, they may pretend that nothing is the matter.

You, and your family as well, may need some time to adjust to the diagnosis before you can begin to deal with cancer in a way that best helps you fight the disease.

When your doctor suspects cancer because of your symptoms, medical history, and/or physical examination he (or the specialist to whom he has referred you) will order the specific diagnostic tests warranted by these preliminary findings. These tests are to enable your physicians to diagnose your illness and to identify its stage.

The following diagnostic tests are usually done prior to any treatment. Some of them may be repeated at intervals to measure your response to treatment. Some may be done after you have completed treatment.

LABORATORY TESTS

Many laboratory tests are rather simple (from the patient's point of view) but can nevertheless reveal a great deal of information. Blood tests, as well as stool and urine samples, are easily obtained and can be examined in a laboratory for any evidence of abnormality.

Hemoccult, or guaiac, tests search for traces of blood in the stool, which is the earliest warning sign for cancer of the rectum or colon. Samples of stool are taken by the patient at home after a few days on a restricted diet, and placed on a specially treated paper, like a slide or tab. This paper is then returned to the doctor, where it is analyzed in a laboratory. You can purchase a similar "do-it-yourself" kit in drugstores, but readings are not always accurate, according to some experts.

Cytology, which deals with the examination of cells, is performed by obtaining a smear of tissue or cells from your body. These cells are then stained with dye and evaluated for cancer and other abnormalities. A pathologist examines the slide under a microscope, after which he or your own doctor may send it to other pathologists for their opinions. Examples of cytological tests are the Papanicolaou (Pap) smear (which can detect early cervical cancer), sputum tests (which can help detect cancer of the lung), and scrapings from the mouth (which can help detect oral cancer).

These laboratory tests provide a good beginning to the full diagnostic procedure and staging. If suspicious cells are found, further studies—such as the following diagnostic tests—are scheduled.

BODY IMAGING

The term *body imaging* refers to tests involving such techniques as X rays, nuclear scans, ultrasound, and thermography, all of which give a picture of various organs and other parts of your body. These tests are performed in a radiologist's office or in the radiology or nuclear-medicine department of a hospital. A radiologist is a physician who specializes in various kinds of body imaging, most of which make use of radioactive substances. Specialists in nuclear medicine are trained in internal medicine, pathology, and radiology, as well as nuclear medicine, and may specialize in many of the newer nuclear imaging tests, as described on pages 21–23. All body imaging should be done under the supervision of a physician who is board-certified in radiology, nuclear medicine, or, in some instances, such specialties as a gynecology, gastroenterology, or urology. The tests are usually performed or administered by nonphysicians trained in the use of the equipment they handle. These well-trained health-care professionals are known as technicians or technologists. For reasons of uniformity, we will refer to all such nonphysicians as technologists. The *interpretation* of these imaging tests is *always performed by a physician.*

You have probably at some time had the conventional chest X ray, sometimes referred to as a "chest plate." This is an X ray that takes a picture of your chest and lungs. It is often done during a regular medical examination and in pre-employment medical examinations. Traditionally, the chest X ray screens for tuberculosis and cancer of the lung. It is the most frequently requested X ray and can give valuable information on conditions of the heart, lungs, gastrointestinal tract, and thyroid gland. Most of the tests performed by a radiologist involve X rays; following are some of the different types you may encounter:

Mammography is the X-ray examination of the breasts. Though the X rays involved are low-dose, it is a powerful tool for detecting breast cancer even before the growth can be felt on examination. If your doctor finds a suspicious bump, skin changes or general lumpiness in the breast, or if you report pain in a breast, he may send you for a mammogram. Mammograms are also done with routine frequency following a mastectomy of the opposite breast. These tests are meant to supplement regular physical breast exams by both the physician and yourself.

Mammograms, like other X rays, reveal the inner structure of the body. The machine uses a cone-shaped device to help position your breast. It touches the breasts on two sides, and although there is some squeezing discomfort, there is no pain. The test is usually performed by a technologist, the X rays are then studied and evaluated by a radiologist, who will send the results to your referring physician. Often, the radiologist will also physically examine your breasts and discuss findings of both the exam and the mammography with you.

Note: Mammograms are widely recommended for screening of *all* women over age thirty-five, even those who show no symptoms and have no history of breast cancer in their families. In 1986 the American Cancer Society recommended the following frequency: between the ages of thirty-five and forty, a woman should have a baseline mammogram; between forty and forty-nine, a mammogram every one or two years (the decision as to whether the test should be annual or biannual is based on individual and family history); and a yearly mammogram after fifty. Because the total amount of radiation absorbed in a mammogram of both breasts should not exceed 2 rads, annual mammograms do not present a risk of overexposure to radiation. When you make your appointment for a mammogram, ask how many total rads the radiologist uses, and if it exceeds 2 rads, go elsewhere.

Tomography is a type of X-ray examination that takes pictures indicating various depths of the body. Unlike conventional X rays, these scans provide three-dimensional information on tissues, rather than just bone.

The procedure is usually referred to as a CAT scan or a CT scan (short for computerized tomographic scanning, computer-assisted tomography, or computerized axial tomography). Computers and X rays are used to take pictures of the body in cross-sectional (front-to-back) "slices," rather than "flat" (head-to-toe) pictures, as in routine X rays. The scan, or picture, appears on a televisionlike screen and can also be printed on photographic paper.

Unlike regular X rays, the CAT scan can actually help determine the size and volume of a tumor. The computer calculates the density of each area, and this density is then recreated on the viewing screen and in photographs. By studying images in sequence, the radiologist builds up a three-dimensional picture of the inner structures, allowing him to estimate with some precision the size, shape, and location of the tumor. The CAT scan's sharp images of such details as blood vessels, fluid compartments, and tissue structure within solid organs permit diagnosis that was previously only available through exploratory surgery.

The machinery used for a CAT scan is huge and awesome to view, but the test is completely painless. You will lie on a table, which is moved into the center of a large ring through which the scan is made. You will hear the sounds of gears and motors as the scanner takes a series of pictures. For each new image, the table will move you into another position.

You may be asked not to eat for several hours prior to the test. Usually, a medication called a contrast medium (a type of dye) is injected into your arm, either by hypodermic needle or, more gradually, from an intravenous bottle. This dye helps to highlight internal structures. It has an iodine base but should not cause any problems unless you are allergic to fish. Before the test you will be asked about this, and if necessary, you will be given antihistamines to prevent an allergic reaction. Occasionally, people with no known allergies have an adverse reaction. The staff in attendance will be prepared to treat this problem if it should occur.

The test is conducted by a technologist highly skilled in the use of the equipment, but the results are evaluated by a radiologist especially trained in "reading" CAT scans. He will discuss the findings with your referring physician.

The CAT does not require hospitalization, and is now available in many communities. If not available in yours, your doctor will locate the nearest medical center where you can have this test.

Some X rays are described as *invasive* tests because they require a contrast substance to be introduced directly into the body. This is done so that the image of a specific area will be outlined and hence stand out clearly for examination.

CAT scans usually make use of dye as a contrast material (as described above), but they can be performed without it. Following are several other invasive tests your doctor may order. Some use air or radioactive material as the contrast substance.

Angiograms, also called arteriograms, visualize vessel structures and arteries leading to various organs. Dye is injected into the appropriate artery, and then an X ray or series of X rays is taken to give the physician information about the organs themselves as well as the arteries and lymph glands. The dye is introduced into the body by means of an injection, usually intravenous (through a vein), or a thin catheter inserted and threaded into an artery. The dye then travels through the bloodstream to a designated area.

Angiograms can be done of legs, kidneys, pancreas, liver, GI tract, brain, and heart. *Cardiac catheterization*, or angiocardiography, visualizes arteries going into the heart; *renal arteriography* can reveal cancer of the kidneys. Dye is injected into arteries that serve the brain and/or spinal cord for an angiogram of the brain. At one time dye was injected into the neck or skull for this test, but today it is introduced through the femoral vein, which is located in the thigh, or through the brachial artery, which is located in the crease of the elbow.

Angiograms are extremely useful for diagnosing lymph-node involvement in cancer. During these tests, called *lymphangiograms*, dye is injected into the lymph channels in the feet, near the big toes. This test is especially useful in the diagnosis of lymphomas and leukemias, as well as in detecting spread of cancer to the lymph system.

In a *venogram*, the dye is injected into the femoral vein to visualize the vena cava (the major vein in the abdomen). This test is useful for diagnosing abnormal masses between lungs and near the abdominal wall.

The dye used in all of the above tests gives you a sensation of heat, sometimes intense, but only during injection. The doctor or technologist will advise you if this is to be expected. It takes time for the dye to reach its destination, so the procedure can take several hours.

To prevent bleeding from the artery used as the site of introduction for an angiogram, you may be required to lie down for a few hours. Thus this test is frequently done on an inpatient basis. Some dyes remain in the body for up to a few months. In these instances, tests may be repeated and changes monitored without reintroduction of new dye.

Statistically, there is little risk involved with most angiograms, although an occasional patient may experience an allergy. Some angiograms, such as those of the brain, pulmonary vessels, and heart chambers, pose a slightly higher risk because of the possibility of stroke, nerve damage, or other complications. Some of these tests have been replaced or supplemented by the newer CAT scans, ultrasound, and nuclear scans (described later). Before you have an angiogram, ask your doctor if it is possible to substitute the newer tests.

Fluoroscopies, sometimes referred to as *flow studies*, also make use of contrast material, charting its progress through a part of the body. The physician watches the contrast move through the body on a machine called a fluoroscope, which looks something like a television screen displaying a "motion-picture X ray." The doctor also takes X-ray pictures providing him with a permanent record of what he has observed on the screen.

A GI *series* makes use of fluoroscopies. These are tests that visualize the entire gastrointestinal system (the organs from mouth to anus). An upper GI series requires the swallowing of barium, a white opaque chemical substance. In a lower GI series, the barium is inserted into the rectum by means of an enema.

You must abstain from ingesting any food or liquids for at least eight hours before an upper GI series. Just before, and at some point during this test, you will be given a liquid barium mixture to drink. The fluoroscope will allow the radiologist or gastroenterologist to watch the barium flow into the digestive system. The barium mixture coats the walls of the upper digestive tract, blocking the X rays, rather than allowing them to pass through it. The upper digestive tract is then revealed as sharply as your bones. Any obstruction or abnormality will be observed because the barium cannot pass through it.

The night before having a lower GI series, you will probably be asked to take a laxative and completely cleanse your colon by means of an enema. You will be told to have a clear-liquid diet at the evening meal prior to the test, and you may be asked not to eat anything the morning of the test. At the radiologist's or gastroenterologist's office, you will be given an enema consisting of a liquid barium mixture. As in the upper GI series, the barium will coat the walls of the lower digestive tract (colon and rectum) blocking X rays and allowing the entire system to be clearly viewed. Air may be pumped into the rectum as well, providing additional contrast.

A GI series is administered by a technologist, but the physician (radiologist or gastroenterologist) will also be there to observe it on the fluoroscope and to decide when to take the X rays for later reference. This test can be done in the doctor's office or in the outpatient department of a hospital.

An *intravenous pyelogram* (IVP) is another example of a flow study, consisting of a series of X-ray pictures. It requires the injection of a dye to outline the bladder, ureters, and kidneys. This test is done in a urologist's or radiologist's office or in the outpatient department of a hospital.

Contrast medium, as described in the above tests, may be either radiopaque (not permitting transmission of X rays) or radiolucent (permitting the transmission of X rays but offering some resistance).

Dyes and barium are examples of radiopaque contrasts. Air is a radiolucent medium. Air may be introduced very simply with the deep breath you take and hold, filling your lungs, during a chest X ray. During other tests (like the lower GI series), air might be introduced by injection, pumping, or other means.

A few of the tests described above (those requiring the injection of dye) carry some element of risk because of immediate adverse allergic reactions. But even so, any responsible physician or radiology department is prepared to successfully overcome any such reactions. Except during pregnancy, X rays in themselves represent minimal risk if they are not indiscriminately repeated. Cancer patients may require many tests, including X rays, so that the doctor can obtain an accurate diagnosis and then, later, follow up the effects of treatment. Most experts agree that the benefits to cancer patients from obtaining accurate information about their disease outweigh any potential risk of radiation exposure.

CAT scans have replaced some angiograms and are safer and more comfortable for the patient. However, these and other newer tests described below are not the answer to *all* diagnostic imaging. Many of the traditional tests are still essential to an accurate diagnosis.

Your physician may send you to a radiologist or to the outpatient department of your local hospital for many of these tests, but other specialists are equipped to do some tests in their offices. For instance, a gastroenterologist can do a GI series, a urologist can do an intravenous pyelogram, and many orthopedists do all their own X rays of bones.

For your safety, as well as for obtaining the most accurate diagnostic results, you should *insist that these X rays be done by either a board-certified radiologist or a specialist in the area that is being imaged.* Too often patients arrive at the oncologist's office with X rays that are not sharp and clear, and they have to go through the process all over again.

It is important that the equipment be regularly inspected (some states post an inspection notice next to it), not emit too much radiation, and give good clear pictures. It would be rather awkward and even impractical to check this after you are in the X-ray room, so when you make an appointment for X rays, ask these questions:

Is the doctor board-certified in either radiology or the specialty being tested? If the answer to this question is negative, go elsewhere. If your personal physician cannot recommend a board-certified radiologist in your community, call your local hospital and ask for a recommendation, or check with the directory of specialists at your local library.

When was the equipment last inspected? Equipment should have been inspected within the last two years.

Before submitting to angiograms and other tests that require contrast dye, ask your doctor if some other newer tests, such as CAT scan or those listed below, could yield the same information. It is possible that your doctor has ordered the older tests simply because the newer ones are not available in your community. Almost all the tests listed below are now widely available, however, so you should not have far to travel to obtain the benefit of the latest and safest diagnostic tests. Ask your doctor if the tests he has ordered are those of choice, not just convenience.

Nuclear Scans make use of a small amount of radioactive-trace compounds sometimes called isotopes but more recently called radionuclides The minute amounts introduced directly into the body, orally or by injection, are called radiopharmaceuticals. They circulate throughout tissues, organs, and organ systems, depending on how they are administered.

Scans are sometimes named to correspond to various body parts. Thus, for instance, bone scans, liver scans, brain scans, and thyroid scans are of those specific body parts.

A *gallium scan*, requiring an injection of a small amount of gallium-67 into the patient's veins, can show rapidly dividing cells and can detect lymph-node involvement. The dye moves slowly through the system, so the test is repeated over a period of a few days. It is not necessary to have additional injections of gallium when these tests are repeated.

The nuclear-scanning machine itself does not emit any radiation. Although the idea of introducing radioactive substances into your body may cause some apprehension on your part, you can be assured that in almost all instances, these nuclear scans expose you to less radiation than does a standard X ray of the same area.

Nuclear scans are especially useful in visualizing organs and regions within organs that cannot be seen on a simple X ray. Tumors stand out particularly well. These procedures are used to study all parts of the body.

A technologist administers the test, but radiologists trained in nuclear radiology or specialists in nuclear medicine interpret them. The tests are neither dangerous nor painful, and the only discomfort experienced may be from holding still on an uncomfortable hard table.

Ultrasound employs high-frequency sound waves to examine position, form, and function of anatomical structures. The procedure is actually called *ultrasonography* (or, sometimes, echography or sonography). A sonogram, echogram, or scan is the record of the test. During this test, a technologist or physician passes a wandlike instrument called a transducer back and forth over the area to be examined. It transmits sound waves and echoes, which are electronically processed and form a fairly detailed picture on a screen. Images from the reflected sound waves are seen on the screen and can be recorded on paper or X-ray film for future reference. Ultrasound can make the important discrimination between a cyst (which contains fluid and semisolid material) and a solid tumor. It cannot tell the difference, however, between benign and malignant tumors.

Ultrasound is especially useful for gathering information about kidneys, thyroid glands, female reproductive organs, lymph nodes, spleen, and pancreas. It can show large breast masses but is *not* an established approach to screening for breast cancer, although it is sometimes used in conjunction with mammography.

Ultrasound does not use radiation, nor does it require any injection. It is completely painless and harmless and can be repeated many times without being injurious to the patient. It can be done on an outpatient basis. A radiologist or other specialist trained in the procedure interprets sonograms.

Thermography makes use of a camera with heat-sensitive film that records the infrared light radiated by the skin. Any temperature differences in body tissues that may indicate an infection or cancer are thus revealed in a sort of "heat picture." The images of the thermogram appear on a televisionlike screen in various colors, each of which represents a different degree of heat. The value of this test in cancer diagnosis has not yet been fully determined. It was once thought to be useful in breast-cancer screening, but as of 1986 the National Cancer Institute and the American College of Radiology no longer recommend it for that purpose.

Nuclear magnetic resonance (NMR) is a new noninvasive technique that, like the CAT scan, produces a three-dimensional, cross-sectional body image.

The NMR scanner produces visual images even more detailed than the CAT scan. Patients are not exposed to any radiation in this test; instead, radio waves and a magnetic field delineate the tissues. The test is completely safe and painless, and the only complaint patients have is that it is even noisier than the CAT scan.

Because the NMR is such a sensitive device, it can detect dead or degenerating cells, obstruction of blood flow, and subtle chemical changes in lesions that may precede gross physical changes. The images provide information about function as well as structure. Experts predict that it will eventually be very important in cancer diagnosis and staging.

As of the mid-1980s it is being used in some major university hospitals, but because of the great expense involved, it may be some time before these machines are widely available.

ENDOSCOPIES

An endoscope is the general term for a rigid or flexible tubular viewing instrument that is inserted through the mouth, rectum, vagina, urethra, or other natural opening in the body. It permits a physician to look for abnormalities and, with the aid of a cutting attachment or a small brush, to collect cell or tissue samples for examination in the laboratory by a pathologist. It can also be inserted through an incision into the body. Many of the newer endoscopes are fiber-optic instruments, which have a lighted mirror-lens system attached to a flexible tube. During some endoscopies, an X ray is taken, or a picture is relayed to a viewing screen. Videotapes are sometimes made for further evaluation.

There are many varieties of endoscopic instruments. The ending -*scopy* means "looking into." Thus, the bronchoscope, inserted through the nose or mouth, is used to look into and examine bronchial tubes and lungs. The colonscope, inserted into the rectum, permits viewing of the full length of the large intestine, scanning the entire colon. The laparoscope is used to view the abdomen, cystoscope the bladder, protoscope the anus and rectum, sigmoidoscope the lower part of the intestine, and the upper GI endoscope the duodenum, pancreas, esophagus, and stomach. All such endoscopies may involve removing tissue samples as well as viewing.

Endoscopies are excellent diagnostic tests and often permit the physician to diagnose suspected tumors that once could be identified only during a major surgical procedure. For instance, a majority of colorectal (colon or rectum) cancers can be discovered through colonscopy *before* symptoms appear, and then surgery can be done early enough to effect a total cure.

An endoscopic procedure may be uncomfortable, but it need not be painful. Sedation, when necessary, is administered by injection, and the surface area where the scope is passed is sprayed with a surface anesthetic. This minimizes discomfort, and prevents gagging if the scope has to be passed down the throat.

Preparations and procedures vary according to the specific test. If you require intravenous sedation, you may become drowsy, so if it is necessary to drive, you should have someone along to accompany you home. Recuperation time also varies according to the procedure, but in most instances you will be back to your usual routine by the next day.

These tests are usually performed in the outpatient department of a hospital, but some specialists may do them in the office. Gastroenterologists, gynecologists, and urologists are among the specialists who do various endoscopies. Occasionally, your physician may want you to stay overnight in the hospital prior to, or following, an endoscopy.

Although these procedures are quite routine, an occasional complication can arise. Organs can be perforated, but rarely does this occur when the endoscopy is performed by a specialist who has had considerable training and experience. You have every right to ask the doctor who is going to do it if he does the procedure regularly.

BIOPSIES

A biopsy is the removal and microscopic examination of suspected tissue or body fluid. A biopsy can provide the definitive diagnosis of cancer, and at one time it was the *only* way to do so. It is no longer necessary to perform a biopsy in *every* instance of suspected cancer, because some of the diagnostic tests described above can give the same answer.

It is important that a biopsy be done by a physician who is well trained and experienced, so that sufficient tissue or fluid is removed. Proper preparation and examination of the biopsied tissue are equally important, and this is the responsibility of both the physician who removes the tissue or fluid and the pathologist who examines it. Contrary to some popular misconceptions, this procedure, when done properly, does not cause the cancer to spread.

To prepare tissue for examination, it is thinly sliced and mounted on slides that are dyed to highlight certain areas. These slides are examined under a microscope by a pathologist. When fluid has been removed from the body, the pathologist examines it by way of chemical analysis.

Some biopsies can be done in a doctor's office or in the outpatient department of a hospital. Others must be done in the hospital. The physician makes the decision based on various factors including the location of the suspected cancer and your general health. Two methods of slide preparation and several kinds of biopsies are described below.

A *permanent section* is prepared by putting tissue in chemical solutions and adding certain dyes which result in highly accurate and detailed information that is permanently preserved. It can be sent to a pathologist in another medical institution for a second opinion and interpretation. A *frozen section* is prepared quickly, in a matter of fifteen to twenty minutes, and this also reveals important information. Tissue sections are hardened by quick freezing, then sliced and studied under the microscope. This procedure results in thicker slices than in the permanent section. These slides must be "read" immediately; they cannot be preserved and sent to another pathologist. Complete analysis is not possible.

Frozen sections are usually performed when a patient is having an incisional or excisional biopsy (see below) in an operating room. The advantage of a frozen section is that in some instances, if the patient has agreed beforehand, a decision to proceed with further surgery can be made while a patient is still under anesthesia. A major disadvantage of relying on a frozen section is that it cannot always determine the exact type of cancer. Interpretations made from examining frozen sections of some organ specimens are more accurate than others, but even so, occasionally a frozen section from a tumor appears to be benign but is *not*. Patients and families celebrate the good news, only to find out a few days later that the permanent sections have revealed the presence of cancer.

Incisional biopsy. An incision is made into the body to remove a portion of the tumor along with adjacent tissue. Occasionally, two or more parts of a tumor are removed, to be certain that representative samples are being examined. The doctor makes a small incision in the skin if the tumor is easily felt on or near the surface. He can perform this procedure under local anesthesia either in his office or in the hospital. Biopsy of a tumor that is deep inside the body may require general anesthesia and must be done in an operating room in the hospital.

Excisional biopsy. This is actually a surgical procedure that involves the removal of the entire tumor.

If a mole, small lump, or thickening on an arm or leg is near the surface, or if the tissue or tumor is small or precancerous, the doctor will probably choose to remove it completely.

If a tumor or growth is causing an obstruction, it may be removed regardless of size.

Your physician will discuss the details of the planned excisional biopsy with you prior to the procedure. Depending on the size, nature, and location of the tumor, an excisional biopsy may be done in a doctor's office, in a hospital outpatient operating room, or may require a hospital stay.

Needle biopsy (or aspiration). There are two kinds of needle biopsies: fine-needle and wide-needle. A very fine, thin needle can aspirate (extract) fluid from an organ or other part of the body. Samples of the fluid are then analyzed. A wide-needle biopsy can make use of a small cutting instrument, which is inserted through the needle, or the needle can be twisted to cut away a small sample of tissue.

A local anesthetic is sufficient to perform most needle biopsies, and they are frequently done in the doctor's office or in the outpatient department of the hospital.

A needle biopsy into solid tissue can sometimes give a false result because the needle can miss the cancerous cells. However, this procedure is a useful early step in the diagnostic process because if the findings *do* indicate cancer, you may not require any further biopsies during the evaluation and workup period.

Some aspiration biopsies are very specific and yield necessary and important information.

Bone-marrow aspirations. Bone marrow is the soft, spongy material at the center of the bone that produces many of the important components of blood, such as white blood cells, red blood cells, and platelets. Bone-marrow aspiration is a biopsy in which a long, hollow needle is inserted into the chest or hip bone of a prone patient. A sample of the marrow is suctioned out to send to the pathologist for analysis.

This test is done when the physician suspects leukemia or other cancers that originate in the bone marrow. It is also done to detect if cancer has spread to the marrow from another location. Hematologists (physicians who specialize in conditions of blood and blood-making tissues) are trained to do this test. It may be performed in either the doctor's office or the hospital. It is somewhat uncomfortable and can cause brief pain.

The following procedures are used both for diagnosis and for administering medication or removing accumulated fluid that is causing discomfort.

A *spinal tap* (also known as a lumbar puncture) is done to remove fluid from the spine, revealing information about the nervous system (brain and spinal cord).

In this test, the doctor—usually a neurologist (a physician who specializes in disorders of the nervous system)—inserts a needle through the space between the vertebrae (backbones) to remove about one to two teaspoons of spinal fluid. It is not usually painful, but you may experience uncomfortable pressure as the needle is inserted.

This procedure can be done in a physician's office if provisions can be made for the patient to lie prone for four to eight hours after it is done. This will help to avoid a headache. The patient should also be observed for any temporary adverse neurological reactions.

Thoracentesis (also known as a pleural tap) is a procedure in which fluid is removed from the pleural space (the area surrounding the lungs). The patient sits over a pillow with arms crossed. Local anesthetic, which may sting, is inserted from your back into the pleural space. Then the doctor uses a long needle with a syringe attached to remove the fluid, which is then examined for evidence of cancer cells or other abnormalities. This test is uncomfortable and you may experience some pressure, but little or no pain. The doctor can perform it in his office or in the outpatient department of a hospital. It is often done by a physician or surgeon who specializes in chest diseases but can be done by others who have experience with the technique. The procedure is also done to withdraw accumulated fluid from the pleural space and to administer medication.

Paracentesis is a procedure similar to thoracentesis; here, fluid is removed from a body cavity. It is usually done to remove excess fluid from the abdomen.

Endoscopic biopsy. During an endoscopy (see pages 23–24), a physician can remove small tissue samples for analysis. Endoscopic biopsies have made it possible to obtain diagnoses that were once possible only during major surgical procedures. These procedures can often be done in the doctor's office, but in some instances they may be done in the outpatient department of a hospital or you may be required to stay overnight there.

ELECTROENCEPHALOGRAM

This test is most commonly known as an EEG. It is a painless procedure that takes one or two hours of waking time. If your doctor has also ordered a "sleep EEG," it will take an extra hour.

The test measures electrical activity of various parts of the brain and is useful in diagnosing brain tumors and other abnormalities.

For this test, you will be seated or lying down in a neurologist's office or a special department of the hospital. Nineteen to twenty-one electrodes will be attached to your head with paste or needles. The paste is somewhat messy; if needles are used, you will experience a feeling similar to having your hair yanked quickly. The test is otherwise painless. The electrodes pick up electricity from your brain; they do *not* give off any electricity. The electrical activity is passed on to a machine that translates the information into lines on graph paper.

Flashing lights are sometimes placed in front of your eyes, or you may be asked to breathe deeply and quickly for a few minutes to observe changes in the brain waves.

If your doctor has ordered a sleep EEG, you will be given a mild sedative so that you can sleep while the test is being done. If you are able to go to sleep during the test without a sedative, it can be omitted.

A technologist may administer the test, but a neurologist interprets it. If the test is done on an outpatient basis and you are going to receive sedation to sleep, you may remain groggy, so it might be wise to have someone accompany you home.

Costs of Diagnostic Examinations and Tests

Many insurance policies do not pay for regular preventive and routine health care but *do* pay for diagnostic examinations. Most of the diagnostic tests and examinations described here are only done if your physician suspects some abnormality. Thus, most insurance plans, including Blue Cross and Blue Shield, Medicare, and other major-medical policies, will reimburse you in part or completely for the examinations and tests. If you have any questions, call your insurance company.

The Importance of Staging

As we explained in the beginning of this chapter, when cancer is first suspected or diagnosed, the staging process begins. This is the process of evaluating precisely *where* the cancer is located, *if* and *how far it has penetrated*, and the *precise types of cells* that are involved. Cancer cells or tumors are described as either "well differentiated" (which means that they are well structured and likely to be slow growing) or as anaplastic, or "poorly differentiated" (meaning that they have a more chaotic structure and are likely to grow quickly). This diagnosis and evaluation is made by making use of one or more of the diagnostic tests described above. Many of these tests complement, rather than duplicate, each other.

Years ago, as soon as any test verified the diagnosis of cancer, the surgeon removed the tumor and, if possible, the organ. Only *after* surgery was an attempt made to determine the extent of the cancer.

Today, whenever possible, staging is done as part of the diagnostic procedure and continues *after* confirmation of diagnosis but *before* major surgery or treatment. If the cancer has already spread from its site of origin to other parts of the body, a major operation may *not* be the best approach. Radiation or chemotherapy may be more effective. (See Section 2 for a full description of various treatments.) In some instances, radiation or chemotherapy are administered to shrink the tumor and surgery is performed at a later date.

Although different cancers are staged in different ways, the principle remains the same; prior to treatment, every relevant diagnostic tool is used to learn how far the cancer has progressed. Based on this information, the most effective treatment plan can be instituted. Another reason for staging is to establish a "baseline" so that your physicians can carefully monitor you and know if you are responding favorably to treatment. Tests are frequently repeated during the course of treatment to measure your response to it.

Some cancers *cannot* be definitively diagnosed without exploratory surgery. On the basis of many tests, including physical examination and an endoscopy, your physician may suspect an ovarian or intestinal tumor. If the tests do not yield sufficient information, it is often necessary to perform a surgical procedure that involves an incision through the abdomen so that the surgeon can inspect the ovaries and/or interior of the abdomen. At the same time, he looks for any hard areas (called nodules) and carefully explores any lymph nodes in the area for evidence of cancer. Based on these observations, and sometimes a frozen section, further surgery may be performed. No physician would want to subject a patient to abdominal surgery twice—once to "look" and another time to "remove"—unless absolutely necessary. Even if the suspicious tumor turns out to be benign, exploratory surgery is a major operation. In the interest of the best possible medical care, and in response to patient concerns, physicians try to get the most information possible *without* doing surgery. The very sophisticated diagnostic techniques described earlier have made this possible in instances when only a few years ago surgery was essential for diagnosis and staging.

Your cancer has now been diagnosed and staged. Hopefully, you feel confident that you have found yourself a competent, knowledgeable, and experienced cancer specialist and that you have been told the extent of your disease. Ask your doctor to tell it to you in an understandable fashion, rather than by simply stating the number of the stage.

Your doctor will recommend a course of treatment to you. At this point you may wish a second opinion. If you seek one, be sure that all records of your tests are sent to this doctor before your consultation. You may also—though it is not necessary—wish to ask your physician to submit your case to a tumor board. This is an official committee in a hospital or community composed of physicians including medical, radiation, and surgical oncologists; pathologists; and sometimes other health professionals. They review cases of cancer in their hospital as well as those sent to them from elsewhere, and make recommendations concerning further diagnosis or treatment.

The full impact of the diagnosis may begin to affect you at this time. Reactions vary, and as Chapter 16 discusses in depth, coping mechanisms also vary.

No matter how overwhelmed you may feel, you should begin

treatment as soon as your doctor suggests. Remember: Early treatment is essential for obtaining the best results. There may be some difficult days ahead, but knowing that the planned treatment—surgery, radiation, chemotherapy, or a combination of these and other treatments—is the right one can give you strength, hope, and optimism.

Section Two

TREATMENTS FOR CANCER

Chapter 4
Surgery

Cancer is treated today in several ways, most often by surgery, radiation, and chemotherapy, each of which I'll discuss in this section.

Many forms of cancer can be treated successfully by surgery alone, especially if the tumor has not spread from its place of origin. Even when surgery alone effects a cure, and you require no further treatment, you should have regular medical checkups for the rest of your life.

Cancer of the colon, breast, and lung are some of the cancers in which surgery is the usual treatment—though in some instances, radiation or chemotherapy may be preferable. Very often, radiation and/or chemotherapy follow surgery; they are then referred to as *adjuvant therapy*, or combined therapy. In Chapter 9 I will discuss specific types of cancer, their symptoms and usual treatments.

What Is Surgery?

Surgery is that branch of medicine concerned with the art and practice of treating diseases, injuries, and deformities by operation, using manipulation or instruments. Some surgery is very minor. The removal of a splinter from a hand or the application of splints and bandages is sometimes described as minor surgery. The term *major surgery* usually describes procedures such as the removal of a large tumor or the amputation of a limb part. *Conservative surgery* aims to avoid mutilation or removal of parts of the body. Describing surgical procedures as major or minor depends upon your outlook. Someone once commented, "An operation is minor when the doctor performs it, but it's major when *he* is the patient."

Some patients resist surgery because they believe that exposing the cancer to air, as well as the procedure itself, will hasten the spread of the disease. Competent surgeons today are careful not to handle polyps, tumors, or tissues prior to removal, so as to avoid infection and the spread of cancer cells, if any are present, throughout the body. There is no evidence, however, to support the belief that exposing cancer to the air can cause spreading, yet this myth persists, preventing many people from seeking early treatment and surgery for a *primary* (original) tumor.

Who Performs Surgery?

Anyone who has graduated from medical school and is licensed to practice medicine can, by law, perform surgery. However, most hospitals only allow minor surgery to be performed by a physician who is not trained in surgery.

More than half of all surgeons in the United States are board-certified in the field, and you should have your surgery performed by one of these surgeons. Board-certified general surgeons are qualified to perform all forms of surgery, although most of them specialize in treating the abdominal area. You should be certain that any surgeon who operates on you is experienced in doing the particular procedure you will be undergoing.

In addition to general surgeons, there are other board-certified surgical specialties and subspecialties. Many of these surgeons have had training in general surgery as well as in their chosen subspecialty.

Orthopedists treat diseases and perform surgery on the skeletal system, bones, joints, and ligaments.

Urologists treat diseases and perform surgery on the ureter, bladder, prostate gland, and male genital organs. They also operate on kidneys, but diseases of the kidney are usually treated by physicians who specialize in internal medicine with a subspecialty in nephrology.

Neurosurgeons operate on the central nervous system, including the brain, spinal cord, and peripheral nerves. Diseases of the central nervous system are treated by neurologists.

Thoracic surgeons perform surgery on the heart, lungs, and esophagus.

Plastic surgeons perform skin grafts, repair tendons and nerves, and do surgery that alters, replaces, or restores visible portions of the body.

Obstetricians and *gynecologists* attend to childbirth, treat female genital disorders, and perform operations on the female reproductive organs; *gynecology oncologists* specialize in treating cancer of the female reproductive organs.

Ophthalmologists treat diseases of the eyes and optical structures, and perform surgery on that area.

Dermatologists treat diseases of the skin and scalp and perform surgery on those areas.

Colon and Rectal surgeons perform surgery on the intestinal tract, rectum, anal canal, and perianal area. However, general surgeons also do this surgery very competently.

Otolaryngologists, also known as ENT physicians, treat diseases and perform surgery on the ear, nose, and throat and the air tubes to the lungs and neck region. Some of these surgeons specialize in head and neck cancer.

Some surgeons in the above specialties have chosen to focus their practice on treating cancer patients, and belong to various organizations of surgeons specializing in cancer. As discussed on pages 7–8, there is no board certification in surgical oncology.

Where Will the Surgery Be Done?

Surgery can be done in a doctor's office or clinic, or in the operating room of a hospital. The offices of some surgeons are equipped to handle certain surgical procedures that do not require an overnight stay. Skin cancers, for instance, are often removed in the doctor's office even if they are serious and have the potential of spread. Many hospitals have outpatient or ambulatory-care operating rooms for surgery from which people can recover briefly (within a few hours) and go home.

Most operations, however, will necessitate hospitalization. When you learn where your doctor plans to operate on you, be sure that the hospital is accredited by the Joint Commission on Accreditation of Hospitals (JCAH). (To be accredited, a hospital is inspected by members of the medical profession and its staff answers a detailed questionnaire. Medicare payments will not be given to a hospital without accreditation, nor will interns and residents receive credit for training there.) Your doctor, the hospital itself, or your local department of health or medical society can provide you with that information. If the hospital is *not* accredited by the JCAH, ask you. doctor if he works in another hospital that is accredited.

What Is the Goal of Surgery?

Cure or longtime survival is the goal of most surgical procedures for cancer. But there are several other reasons for undergoing surgery. Some surgical procedures are for diagnosis only (as discussed in the section on biopsies, in Chapter 3). Other procedures are for palliation—that is, to eliminate or reduce pain or discomfort.

Most surgical procedures can be grouped into these categories: preventive, specific, radical, and palliative surgery. The type of surgery you will have depends on several factors: type of cancer, size of tumor, location, boundaries of the disease, and your general condition.

PREVENTIVE SURGERY

Just as it sounds, preventive surgery is performed to prevent the development of cancer. Polyps in the colon or rectum, cysts in the breast, moles or growths on the skin, and growths on the larynx are frequently removed because they represent precancerous conditions that may later develop into cancer. Although these growths are benign (noncancerous), experience tells your doctor that such a growth frequently precedes the development of a malignant (cancerous) growth.

Many myths surround cancer and cancer treatment, and at one time people thought that those who frequently developed noncancerous cysts, moles, and polyps never really got cancer. *But this is not so.* These noncancerous conditions are frequently a precursor of cancer, and indeed, people with a history of rectal polyps have a higher-than-average risk of developing cancer in the rectum or colon.

Some skin lesions, which are visible abnormalities of tissues, are related to chronic exposure to sunlight and may develop into cancer. We will discuss this in more detail in Chapter 9.

If your doctor tells you that a growth or lesion is *not* cancer, only precancerous, but is firm in wanting to remove it, *heed his advice.* The objective of preventive surgery is just as it sounds: to prevent cancer from developing where the potential for it is great.

SPECIFIC AND RADICAL SURGERY

Specific and radical surgery are the most common kinds of surgery for cancer.

Specific surgery is done when a tumor is present, has not spread, and can be completely removed. In specific surgery, the aim is to remove all the tissues that are believed to be malignant. It is the treatment of choice for many cancers, and sometimes no other treatment is required. Cure has been achieved. In other instances, further treatment—such as radiation and/or chemotherapy—is necessary.

Radical surgery is treatment intended to cure, not just palliate. In this way, it is really the same as specific surgery.

However, this term is most often used to describe definitive, extreme treatment, consisting of the removal of the entire organ and adjacent malignant tissue. This kind of surgery can be limited or extensive, and may be followed immediately or at a later date by chemotherapy or radiation. Sometimes chemotherapy or radiation is used first to shrink the tumor to a more manageable and operable size.

The decision as to whether to perform surgery prior to, instead of, or following chemotherapy or radiation is based on many conditions including type of tumor, location, and other individual factors, such as the general health of the patient. You will find more information on this in Section 3, where I'll describe different types of cancers.

When the surgeon removes the tumor, he also often removes the lymph nodes in the area near the tumor. This is done for two reasons: to perform a biopsy on the nodes (to determine if they are harboring malignant cells) and to determine if postoperative chemotherapy or radiation is indicated.

PALLIATIVE SURGERY

Palliative surgery is surgery that is designed to relieve or reduce discomfort or pain. Its purpose is not to produce a cure. Palliative surgery can also correct complications developing from cancer. There are many palliative surgical procedures. Sometimes an obstruction is removed; other times specific nerves are cut or an incision is made into the spinal cord to eliminate pain caused by a tumor.

Certain hormone-producing glands are often removed if the particular cancer is dependent on hormones for growth. Examples of these kinds of cancers are breast and prostate. Hormone dependency is determined by various hormonal-receptor tests, which pathologists perform on tissue that is removed during biopsy. The removal of hormone-producing glands is often defined as palliative, but it can also produce a cure or long remission, the disappearance of signs and symptoms of cancer.

Palliative surgery may be done strictly for comfort and may or may not bear a relation to the progression of disease; neither your nor your family should be alarmed if your doctor recommends it.

OTHER SURGICAL TECHNIQUES

Although most surgery is done with a scalpel or variation thereof, other methods have been developed that have a definite place in cancer treatment and cure. Indeed, their use seems to be growing as new techniques are strengthened and more surgeons are trained in their use. *Cauterization*, for instance, is the destruction of tissue with an electric current, a heated instrument, or a chemical substance.

Chemosurgery

The direct application of strong chemicals, such as zinc chloride, onto certain skin cancers is called chemosurgery. The chemical remains on the skin for up to twenty-four hours, during which time it kills the cancerous cells. The cells are then removed and examined under a microscope. The procedure can be repeated until all cancer cells have been removed. When the tissue seen under the microscope is normal, it is determined that enough has been removed. This procedure is known as a fixed-tissue technique.

In another similar but newer procedure, called the fresh-tissue technique, the suspected area is cut out and examined microscopically. The procedure is repeated as often as necessary until the lesion is completely eradicated. Frequently the tumor can be totally removed in a single office or clinic visit.

Chemosurgery is useful for some skin cancers on or to the side of the nose, and in recurring skin cancers in which it is difficult to determine the precise borders. This surgery can usually be done in an office or clinic.

The concept of chemosurgery is excellent, but it is very difficult to do, because of the risk of removing too much tissue. It is not a routine procedure, and only those physicians, usually dermatologists, who have been very highly trained in this technique should do chemosurgery. It is useful only when the cancers are easily accessible.

Cryosurgery

Cryosurgery—whose root, *cryo*, means "icy cold" or "frost" in Greek—is a form of surgery that makes use of subzero temperatures (down to −160°C) to destroy tissue such as cancer cells and tumors. In one form of cryosurgery, solid carbon dioxide or liquid nitrogen is applied to a growth with a sterile cotton-tipped applicator. A blister then forms, which is followed by necrosis (death) of the tissue. The procedure can be repeated if necessary.

In other forms of cryosurgery, a freezing chemical is circulated through a metal probe, which is then applied to the tumor or cancerous cells. The tissues freeze when they adhere to the cold metal of the probe. The cell membranes then burst, killing the cells, which are then discarded or absorbed by the body.

Cryosurgery is done in a doctor's office, clinic, or operating room and is used to treat some precancerous growths, very small skin cancers, rectal tumors, and tumors of the head and neck. It is not suitable or effective for all cancers. Dermatologists usually perform cryosurgery on skin cancers. Other specialists also use the technique.

Electrosurgery

Electrosurgery makes uses of surgical instruments that operate on high-frequency current. In *electrocoagulation*, the surgeon uses a needle or snare to destroy tissue. This technique is sometimes referred to as electric cautery or galvanocautery. It is used to treat some cancers of the skin, mouth, and rectum.

Electrodesiccation, also called fulguration, is another form of electrosurgery. Here, tissue is destroyed by burning with an electric spark. It is suitable for elimination of small superficial growths and as an aid in curettage, a procedure in which material is scraped and removed from an organ, cavity, or other body surface.

Depending on the location of the tumor, electrosurgery is done in a doctor's office, clinic, or hospital operating room.

Laser Surgery

The term *laser* is an acronym for Light Amplification by Stimulated Emission of Radiation. Laser beams are an extremely concentrated source of light which give off so much heat that they destroy anything in their path. They are thousands of times more intense than the most powerful light beams, and can be narrowed and aimed so accurately at cancerous cells, and delivered so speedily, that they destroy only the diseased tissue, without affecting the surrounding healthy areas. The laser is a "no-touch" technique that sterilizes as it works. Currently, lasers are used by general surgeons, urologists, gynecologists, otolaryngologists, and a number of other specialists in cancer surgery. Lasers are also widely used in eye surgery. A significant feature of laser surgery is that it coagulates blood and so controls bleeding. This technique should be performed only by a surgeon especially trained in the technique, preferably a member of the recently formed American Board of Laser Surgery.

THINGS TO CONSIDER BEFORE SURGERY

There are a number of things you should think about and consider before the day of your surgery. Ask your surgeon these questions:

What will be involved in the operation, and what do you hope to achieve? The surgeon should be able to tell you if he hopes to achieve cure (if the diagnosis has already been established) or palliation. Does he feel that this is just a precancerous condition? It is very likely that your surgeon will explain that until he gets a complete pathological report, and the staging is completed (as described on pages 13–30) he cannot tell you if the surgery will achieve cure.

What are the risks involved in this surgery, and do the benefits outweigh the risks? Naturally, you will want to know about the risks of surgery, but in dealing with cancer you sometimes have to take risks, especially if the possible benefits outweigh these risks.

What will happen if I wait awhile, or don't have surgery at all? Sometimes the answer might be "Well, we can just watch it and see." But more often the answer will be "The cancer will spread." Remember, *early treatment*, like early diagnosis, ensures the best chance of cure.

How will I feel after surgery? Your doctor should be able to give you a sense of what you can expect after surgery. Will you have much pain? Will you be able to get up soon? Should you expect nausea, vomiting, gas, soreness, dizziness, weakness, headaches? These effects sometimes follow anesthesia and pass quickly. But they may be the result of the surgery itself. Your doctor should be able to tell you if you can expect to find any tubes (such as urinary catheters or stomach tubes) connected to you following surgery. But remember, since the surgeon may not be sure *exactly* what he will have to do until he actually sees the tumor and the extent of the cancer, he may not be able to fully answer this question.

How long will I have to be in the hospital? Your doctor may not be able to give you a precise answer, because people heal at different rates. The extent of the surgery will also be a factor in the length of your hospital stay. He can probably give you a range of how many days you will be hospitalized.

In some states, Medicare and certain insurance companies pay hospitals a fixed amount of money to treat each patient for a specific illness or surgical procedure. This fixed amount is based on the number of days the average patient spends in the hospital, or on the usual services used, for that illness. This new fixed-fee system, or prospective reimbursement, referred to as "DRGs" (for diagnostic-related groups), may eventually result in hospitals charging patients directly for any hospitalized days and services that exceed the guidelines set down by DRGs.

Will the surgery be temporarily or permanently disabling? Unless your surgery is very minor, your doctor will probably tell you to expect to take some time for convalescence, since you may be tired and weak for a while. But in all likelihood, you will feel stronger each day, and soon get back to your usual activities. Your surgeon will be able to tell you about how soon you will be able to do such things as drive a car, do household chores, go back to work, lift something heavy, and resume sexual activities. Don't be afraid to ask specific questions about these and any other activities you feel might be affected.

In most instances you will function normally after convalescing from the removal of part or all of a diseased breast, lung, kidney, uterus, thyroid or prostate. Some surgical procedures in which part or all of the bladder or colon are removed may affect daily functioning because the surgeon may have to create a new outlet for urine or bowel movements. These procedures are described in the chapters on those particular cancers.

After certain surgical procedures, you may need some physical-rehabilitation exercises before resuming regular activities. Again, this will be discussed in the chapters on individual cancers.

How much will all this cost? Ask the surgeon about his fee, and then contact your insurance company to find out how much of this fee will be reimbursed. Unless you have a major-medical policy, the insurance company may pay only a portion of the surgeon's fee. Some surgeons are willing to accept as payment in full whatever the insurance company will give them. If the fee presents a financial hardship or strain, discuss it with your surgeon or his office manager. He may lower his fee for you or suggest a way that you can pay a portion of it in monthly installments.

If relevant, you should find out if your insurance company will pay hospital costs. Most policies will pay for a semiprivate room (for two or more people), but you may be responsible for certain extra costs. Before your surgery, discuss this with the patient-accounts department of the hospital.

Anesthesiologists are the physicians who see to it that you are asleep or experience no pain during surgery. In many hospitals they send separate bills; their fees are not included in the hospital costs. Ask the surgeon or the patient-accounts department about this policy. If your surgeon has adjusted his fee for you for any reason, your anesthesiologist may also be willing to do so.

Will I have more tests? You will probably be admitted to the hospital at least one day prior to surgery. Blood tests, a chest X ray, and an electrocardiogram (EKG, or ECG) are routinely done before any surgery. Some hospitals request that you have these tests performed as an outpatient anytime up to a week before surgery. Your hospital insurance will pay for required tests performed before admission; this pre-admission testing (PAT) is an efficient way to reduce your hospital stay. Some tests may be done *after* admission. This is an individual matter, and depends on several factors: type of test, hospital policy, and your specific needs. Most tests that are planned will be familiar to you from the chapter on diagnosis.

An EKG will detect any cardiovascular (heart and circulatory) abnormalities. During this test, you lie down on your back and a technologist affixes electrodes to your chest, sometimes with an adhesive gel. Electrical impulses from your heart are transmitted to a recording device that produces a graphic reading, which is later interpreted by a physician. The test is neither uncomfortable nor dangerous. The electricity comes *from* you, not *into* you.

Will I be asked a lot of questions once I'm in the hospital? After you are settled in your hospital room, a physician, physician's assistant, nurse, or perhaps all three (but not at the same time) will talk with you. They will obtain your complete medical history by asking you about childhood and adult illnesses, medical problems, previous surgery, allergies, childbirth, miscarriages, any history of bleeding, and close relatives' medical history.

They will also ask about smoking, drinking, and eating habits, about your occupation, and about other matters which may seem irrelevant to you but are an important part of your entire medical picture. You may be asked questions about where and with whom you live, if you have steps in your home, and if your meals are usually eaten at or away from home. Some of this information may be important in planning your care both in the hospital and after discharge.

A physician or physician's assistant, and possibly a nurse, will perform a basic medical examination, including heart, lungs, and blood pressure. Other examinations will be related to the specific reason for your admission and to planned surgery.

What else will happen before surgery?

Intravenous drip (IV): At some time, either the day before, or the morning of surgery, a doctor or nurse may insert an intravenous needle (IV) into your arm. This is done to facilitate giving you any required drugs during or after surgery. The needle is connected to a plastic tube that is attached to a liquid-filled bottle hanging from a pole above your head. The fluid may consist of normal saline (a simple salt-and-water solution), nutrients, or medication.

The fluid will drip in gradually at a predetermined rate. Don't panic if the bottle seems to be empty; without fluid to force it out, no air can get into your veins. Occasionally the needle may become dislodged from the vein, permitting the fluid to get into surrounding tissue. Although this can cause some swelling and discomfort, it is quickly and easily corrected.

Nothing by mouth (NPO, short for non per os): In all likelihood, you will not be allowed to eat or drink anything beginning twelve hours before the surgery. A sign may be hung over your bed, stating NPO, which stands for Non peros os, meaning "nothing by mouth" in Latin. You may also be given a laxative or enema to empty your colon and prepare it for surgery. These precautions provide for greater safety during anesthesia and surgery, and help to minimize nausea and vomiting after surgery.

Sedative: The night before surgery, you may be given a sedative—either by mouth or by injection—to help you fall asleep. It is often difficult to go to sleep in strange surroundings, and when you are also concerned about surgery, it becomes even more difficult. A sedative will help.

Skin preparation: Before surgery, your skin will be prepared (shaved or scrubbed with antiseptics) near and at the site of the planned surgery. This is to prevent infections.

Urinary catheter: A urinary catheter may be placed in your bladder to drain urine during the surgery and afterward. This device is a hollow, flexible tube designed to be passed through the urethra (the muscular canal through which urine passes from the bladder out of the body). The catheter may be inserted prior to surgery or after you are in the operating room. It will be removed after you are able to urinate on your own.

Nasogastric or stomach tube: If the surgery is to be performed in the stomach area, a nasogastric or stomach tube, which is attached to a pump, may be passed through your mouth or nose into the stomach. This keeps the stomach and bowels empty and free of fluids and gas, and helps to limit nausea and vomiting after surgery.

This tube, like the urinary catheter, may be inserted prior to surgery or after you are in the operating room. Depending on the kind of surgery you have, it will be removed at an appropriate time after surgery, usually after you resume normal bowel movements and can begin eating solid food.

Consent Forms

You will be asked to sign a consent form, which outlines the operation that your doctor has explained he is going to perform. Some consent forms are rather simple and easy to read, but others are so complicated that it seems like you need both a medical and a law degree to understand them. These forms can be rather frightening, because they often list many risks that are extremely rare. The doctor who asks you to sign will explain the form to you and may also ask someone to witness your signature. Consent forms are sometimes presented by a busy hospital intern or resident. Don't let yourself be rushed into signing before your questions are answered to your satisfaction.

The form may request that you agree to surgical procedures that have *not* been planned but could become necessary. For example, during surgery to remove an intestinal obstruction, the surgeon may find it necessary to remove a significant part of your colon. You have the right to refuse to sign such a consent form, but you should know that your doctor may then refuse to operate on you. Many surgeons feel they must have the freedom to do more extensive surgery if, in their opinion, it becomes crucial while the operation is in progress.

ANESTHESIA

The night before your operation the anesthesiologist (a physician trained in the administration of anesthetics and in supervising respiratory and cardiovascular care during and after surgery) or anesthetist (a nurse or other health-care professional with advanced training in the specialty of managing the anesthetic care of patients) will probably come to see you. He will ask you several questions about your medical history, allergies, current medications, and any experiences you have had with anesthesia. He will assure you that you will not feel any pain during surgery, and he will usually ask you whether you prefer to be awake or asleep during the operation. The final decision about the type of anesthesia (as described below) will be made by your surgeon and anesthesiologist and will depend on the kind of operation you are having, and on your physical needs. Your wishes will be taken into consideration.

Anesthesia is usually administered by an anesthesiologist or anesthetist. Some surgeons administer their own local anesthetic injections for minor, superficial surgical procedures. During any lengthy procedure, or where there is even a minor medical risk, someone other than the surgeon must assume full responsibility for monitoring the patient's vital signs (cardiac and respiratory condition) and for giving any necessary intravenous fluids and blood transfusions. This is typically the responsibility of the anesthesiologist or anesthetist.

Types of Anesthesia

Topical anesthesia is sprayed or painted on an area, often instead of, prior to, or in addition to, local anesthesia. It offers some superficial numbing and is used only for very minor procedures.

Local anesthesia is injected directly into the surgical site, completely numbing the area. It is used mostly for minor procedures. You may be familiar with this type if you have had dental work, or have had a deep splinter removed from your hand or foot. Local anesthesia affects only a small area.

Regional anesthesia is in some ways similar to local anesthesia but takes in a much larger area. An anesthetic that serves as a deadening agent is injected to temporarily block the transmission of pain from the site of the surgery. You may also be given a sedative.

Spinal anesthesia is the injection of a drug into the sac around the spinal cord, which is part of the central nervous system. The spinal cord is encased by the spinal column, which forms part of the vertebral column, sometimes known as the backbone. Most of the nerves of the body enter or leave the spinal cord through openings in the vertebrae or the area surrounding it, so spinal anesthesia causes complete loss of feeling in the legs and much of the lower part of the body. This effect will linger for several hours following surgery, and there may be some discomfort when it wears off. You will be sedated prior to spinal anesthesia.

General anesthesia is administered either intravenously or by inhalation or a combination of both. Intravenous anesthesia goes directly into the bloodstream; inhalation anesthesia consists of gasses that are breathed through a mask and travel through the lungs into the bloodstream.

The anesthesiologist or anesthetist will monitor you very carefully while you are under general anesthesia. He will keep a constant check on your blood pressure, as well as all pulmonary and cardiovascular functions. He will replace body fluids and blood as necessary. People are often concerned that they will awaken in the middle of their operation. Be assured that this does not happen. General anesthesia can be light or deep; you will be given just enough to keep you completely asleep during your entire operation.

Will I Have a Blood Transfusion?

Loss of blood occurs during some surgical procedures, so all operating rooms are prepared to give a patient blood if it should become necessary. Blood banks and hospitals today are extremely cautious about matching blood type and being certain that any donated blood is free from diseases such as hepatitis and Acquired Immune Deficiency Syndrome (AIDS), but some recent studies suggest that blood transfusions be given *only* when absolutely necessary.

This new attitude has arisen because of findings showing that the immune system in some patients who had blood transfusions during surgery was weakened. Such weakening can hasten recurrence of disease. The theory behind these findings is that even in closely matched blood, proteins in the donor's and recipient's blood do not constitute an exact match. Foreign proteins introduced into the recipient's system can adversely affect his immune system.

You may wish to discuss this with your surgeon prior to surgery.

AFTER SURGERY

When the surgery is completed, you may go to a recovery room or surgical intensive-care unit before returning to your own hospital room.

A recovery room is a sort of way-station between the operating room and the regular hospital room. Nurses with special training monitor postoperative patients' vital signs and make sure that they are awake and able to respond before sending them back to their room.

A surgical intensive-care unit provides the same care as a recovery room but uses the latest in high-technology monitoring equipment. The unit has specialized nursing care and sophisticated methods of supporting a patient if any serious problems related to breathing, circulation, other vital functions arise.

When you first awake from surgery, particularly if you have had general anesthesia, you may feel confused and "spaced out." There may be a number of rubber or synthetic (plastic) tubes coming out of your incisions, an IV dripping liquids into your arm, and a catheter removing urine from your bladder. Sterile bandages and dressings may be covering your incision. All of this is fairly standard and will be removed in good time.

You will return to your hospital room when you no longer require constant monitoring. You will be encouraged to cough after surgery to keep your lungs expanded. This prevents the small air sacs in your lungs from collapsing, which can result in pneumonia. And you will probably be urged to get out of bed before *you* think you are ready. All this pushing may seem heartless, but it is done to hasten your recovery.

After the anesthesia wears off, most people experience some discomfort or pain. The amount of pain varies according to the type and location of surgery. People experience pain differently, but pain *can* be managed, and it is unnecessary for anyone to suffer after surgery. Today's pain medications and dosage plans work to alleviate pain yet still leave you alert and aware of your surroundings. Your surgeon will leave orders with the nurses for you to have pain medication (pills or injections). If pain medication is offered to you, take it *before* the pain becomes intense. It is much easier to prevent pain than it is to relieve it. Sometimes the surgeon leaves the orders "P.R.N." meaning you may take pain medication as often as needed. Other times, the orders may be very specific as to timing. But if you are having a great deal of pain, speak up. Relief is always available. See Chapter 13 for more information on pain management.

Follow-up

The surgeon will tell you (and if he doesn't, ask him) what he found during your surgery. These findings will be based on his own observations, a frozen section, and, sometime later, the permanent section (see Chapter 3).

During your hospitalization you will probably see your medical oncologist as well as the surgeon. Both doctors will advise on the need for further treatment, based on the surgeon's findings and the pathology reports. *If you have not yet seen a medical oncologist, this is the time to be sure to have a consultation.*

Your surgeon may have given you the good news that "we got it all out—you're absolutely clean." That is good news indeed, but you should still be sure to have a medical-oncology consultation, either while you are in the hospital or as soon as you are discharged. Too often, "We got it all out" means "We got everything out we could see," but some malignant cells may have shed into the blood or lymph system. In such an event, the cancer may recur at a later date. Although most surgeons agree that a consultation with a medical oncologist is a wise decision, there are a number of otherwise competent surgeons who still believe that surgery is the major (and almost exclusive) weapon against cancer and are resistant to further treatment for their patients. See a medical oncologist anyway, even if it is only to be reassured that no further treatment is necessary.

Other health professionals. Nurses play a very important part in your care in the hospital and will also teach you how to take care of yourself after you go home. Social workers can help you explore and ventilate your feelings, and collaborate with your physician and nurses to help you plan for discharge. A dietician or nutritionist may consult with you. Aides and technologists will also be part of your health-care team after surgery. In many instances these professionals remain involved in your care after you have gone home. In Section 4, I will discuss this care more fully. And I'll also discuss some of the emotional concerns of everyday living that arise from the diagnosis of cancer, living through cancer and from the surgical procedures themselves.

Chapter 5
Radiation Therapy

Radiation, by definition, is the release of energy from some source, in the form of rays that can pass through certain substances, including skin and flesh. These rays are similar to light and heat rays, but they have much shorter wavelengths and cannot be seen, felt, or smelled. Radiation, as you know, is a feared result of nuclear-bomb explosions and nuclear power-plant accidents, but when it is properly harnessed, as it is for the treatment of cancer, it can be extremely effective.

Radiation therapy, the use of high-energy radiation in the treatment of disease, especially cancer, was first introduced in the early part of this century. But it was another few decades before scientists learned to control dosage and to predict with some accuracy the effects upon both normal and cancerous cells.

Radiation therapy, also known as radiotherapy, X-ray therapy, or cobalt therapy, is a general term to describe many of the various ways that these rays are used to slow, stop, or destroy the growth of cancer cells. Various forms of radiation are the primary treatment for some cancers, and indeed may be the only treatment you will need. Almost half of all cancer patients are treated with radiation. Recent studies have shown that radiation can sometimes be as effective as surgery in treating early, localized tumors. This can save you from disabling or cosmetically undesirable side effects.

Although one or another form of radiation is used for many kinds of cancers, it is especially effective in treating cancers of the prostate, testicles, larynx, and breast, and in early stages of Hodgkin's disease, cancer of the lymph nodes, and many childhood cancers. Radiation can also be effective against cancers of the head and neck, mouth and throat, cervix and uterus, bladder, lung, esophagus, and brain.

Radiation may be given before, after, or instead of surgery. It may be given *prior* to surgery, to shrink a tumor so that it can be more easily removed. Or you may be given radiation *after* surgery, to destroy any remaining malignant cells. Sometimes radiation is directed toward tumors that cannot be reached by surgery or do not respond to drugs. It is also possible that your doctor will want you to have surgery, chemotherapy, and radiation, perhaps in that or some other sequence. Sometimes radiation is used to reduce pressure and bleeding that are causing severe discomfort or pain.

Even when surgery appears to have wiped out your cancer, your surgeon or medical oncologist may recommend that you undergo radiation therapy. This may be because statistical evidence indicates that in situations such as yours some cells tend to shed into adjacent areas. Radiation can destroy these cells, and so is almost like an insurance policy against future trouble.

How Does Radiation Work?

High-intensity, energetic, invisible rays can enter the nuclei of cells and break the strands of genetic material, thus damaging and sometimes killing them. All cells that are exposed to radiation are damaged, but normal, healthy cells recover more quickly than diseased cells. When used on cancer cells, the radiation often kills them, thus shrinking the tumor.

Some cancers are very responsive to radiotherapy; they are described as *radiosensitive*. The cells in these cancers have a rapid rate of division and contain oxygen, which can aid the radiation in its work.

Other cancers are not as responsive to radiotherapy; they are described as *radioresistant*. The cells in these cancers tend to divide slowly, and contain less oxygen. High doses of radiation are required to destroy these cells. Researchers are experimenting constantly with new radiation techniques to have a more potent effect on these cancers.

Repeated small doses of radiation over a period of time allow normal cells to recover more satisfactorily than after a large single dose; thus treatments are often spaced over a period of weeks.

The Different Kinds of Radiation

The early machines, those used in the 1920s and 1930s, used very low power and caused many side effects because the rays were absorbed by the skin, causing adverse skin reactions and great discomfort. At one time, exposure to radiation presented a high health risk. X rays were not well understood, exposure times were too long, and equipment was primitive. It was also more difficult to direct the beams precisely at the tumors, so healthy cells and organs were frequently damaged. Radiotherapy was often reserved for those patients who were "far gone."

Today this has changed. Megavolt, or supervolt, machines produce high-energy rays that can be aimed directly (sometimes from a number of different directions) at the tumor or diseased areas of the body, sparing most of the normal, healthy tissue nearby.

Radiotherapy is not a single type of therapy, nor does it use just one type of machine. For instance, some of the machines, like the Cobalt 60, have radioactive substances placed within them. Other machines, like the linear accelerator or betatron, create their own radioactivity. The radiotherapist will decide which machine is best suited to treat your particular cancer; some machines and techniques destroy shallow tumors near the body's surface; others can penetrate farther, to reach a deep-seated cancer.

If you have radiotherapy, some of the words you may hear are gamma ray, neutron, electron beam, pimeson (or pion), radioactive cobalt, linear accelerator, and betatron. These words refer to various forms of radiation and the machinery used to direct the beams. All the machines are fully shielded, and the radiation is controlled for intensity, duration, and depth.

Most people think of radiation as something that is directed at their tumor from a large machine. However, radiation can also be given internally. A small radiation source may be implanted directly into the body (referred to as a radiation implant) or may be given by intravenous injection or in pill form.

A new technique that is being practiced at certain medical centers is called *intraoperative radiation*. This procedure is performed in the operating room, immediately following surgical removal of all or part of a tumor.

Who Administers Radiotherapy?

The radiotherapy team is led by a physician who is known as a radiotherapist or radiation oncologist, and often includes a radiation physicist (an expert in planning the desired radiation dose), a dosimetrist (who works with the physicist or physician in calculating the dosage), a radiation technologist (who performs many functions, such as delivering the prescribed treatment), and a radiation nurse. Often a social worker is part of the team, there to help patients deal with their feelings about treatment, and to plan transportation and solve other problems that may arise.

Treatment should be planned and supervised only by a specialist in radiation therapy for cancer (a radiotherapist or radiation oncologist; see Chapter 2). The latest, most modern equipment is usually available at major teaching hospitals, but sometimes community hospitals or radiotherapists' offices are also fully equipped. While it may be tempting to "settle" for less than state-of-the-art equipment at your local community hospital because of the convenience of transportation, it is important that you get the best treatment available. If you have any concerns, you can call the radiotherapy department of the nearest comprehensive-care center listed in the appendix to inquire about treatments available near your home.

EXTERNAL RADIATION

Your medical oncologist or surgeon will refer you to the radiotherapist, who will determine the best possible way to give you radiation. If the radiotherapist determines that you should have external radiation (the most common method of administering the treatment), your first visit will most likely involve an·examination, a review of all your medical records, and a discussion of your treatment and expected side effects. You may also have some diagnostic X rays or other tests.

In order to locate the exact area of the body to be treated by radiation, you will be asked to lie down on a large table on which you will be positioned while a series of measurements and X rays, ultrasound or other methods of visualization are done. This is called localization or simulation and may take an hour or more. A radiation technologist will mark the area of the skin to be treated with a special type of waterproof ink or colored dye. This is done so that the radiation can be directed to the same precise area of the body for each treatment. (The marking sometimes stains clothes, so many patients wear old underclothes during the treatment period.) You will be told not to attempt to wash off these marks and, if they should accidentally come off, not to try to redraw them yourself. Many people find the visible markings upsetting even if no one else sees them, because they are a constant reminder of their disease and treatment. It is of some consolation to know that when radiation treatment is completed, the markings will be removed. If radiation is to be directed toward a visible part of the body, such as the head or upper neck, the markings may be made with an "invisible" substance, seen only under a special light. Tattoos may be used instead of marks. They resemble small freckles and provide a permanent record that is useful during time of treatment and in the future.

The physician will tell you the dosage of radiation required, and the number and frequency of treatments. The treatment itself may be as short as a few sessions, or extend daily over many weeks. This plan will be individualized, based on your particular illness and other factors, such as your age and the extent of your disease process. Plan to spend thirty to forty minutes at the radiotherapist's office each visit. You'll need time to wait for the machine to be set up and to change your clothes, as well as to receive treatment.

Although the radiotherapist decides how much total radiation you need, and the amount that you should get at any one session, these may be subject to change. For instance, if you are not tolerating the treatment well, he may decide to give you less radiation at each session, thus prolonging the total duration of therapy. Or he may decide to give it to you only three times a week, instead of the usual five. The response of the tumor may also effect a change in the prescribed dosage or timetable. If you are put on "rest" (no treatment for a few days or longer) because of side effects or some other reason, do not become alarmed. Your doctor knows when this "rest" is appropriate.

For optimum results, it is important that you keep all your treatment appointments; do not skip or cancel them without talking to the radiotherapist. Often the doctor can give you a day or two off, but don't do it on your own. It is tempting, especially when you are tired, the weather is bad, or you just feel like a day off, to "play hookey." Don't yield to the temptation; instead, promise yourself a reward—a special treat, a frivolous purchase, or a vacation—at the end of the treatment.

You will probably not have to stay at the hospital for external radiation. Most people have this therapy on an outpatient basis, although in some instances a patient may be hospitalized for part or all of the treatments. If you are an outpatient, you will probably need to make daily visits for your treatment. If transportation to and from radiation therapy presents a financial or logistical problem, you may be able to obtain assistance from community organizations such as a local church or synagogue, Rotary Club, Red Cross, or the American Cancer Society. The social-work department at your doctor's hospital may be able to make some suggestions.

Treatment sessions. Prior to the treatment, you will be asked to remove your clothes and change into a hospital gown. The technologist will place you in a precise position on the treatment table. You will have to lie still during the treatment, but except for some discomfort from lying on the hard table, you should experience no pain. Bands, metal bars, sandbags, pillows, or plaster casts may be used to hold you in place during the treatment. A large machine that looks somewhat like an X-ray machine will be positioned above you. A light will shine from it onto the area of your body that is to be radiated. The technologist will leave the room, just as he usually does when you have an X ray. This is to avoid his exposure to radiation. Although you may *feel* as if you have been deserted, you will be carefully monitored by means of a closed-circuit television monitor or through a window. An intercom will permit two-way communication between you and the technologist. Radiation itself makes no noise, but some of the machines make a loud clicking or whirring sound. The technologist will tell you when to expect this.

The treatment time depends on the amount of radiation given and the machine used, but the time for the actual therapy generally ranges from one to ten minutes. Delays in waiting for treatment are sometimes unavoidable, so you will probably have to wait for a while in the waiting room. Sometimes a nurse or social worker organizes discussion groups for patients where your questions and concerns can be addressed. Many patients like to bring something to read or do while they are waiting. One patient said she finally carried through on last year's New Year's resolution. Over a six-week period, during the time she waited for treatments, she put her address book, Christmas card list, and family birthday list in order. Other patients come with friends or family members and use the time to chat. The waiting rooms are safe and do not pose a risk of radiation, although many radiotherapy centers advise pregnant women not to accompany patients on a regular basis.

Am I Radioactive After Receiving External Radiation? Absolutely not. No radiation is emitted from the machine once it is turned off or from the patient. Yet many people worry about this and are fearful of close contact with loved ones. Other people are afraid to go near patients receiving treatment. Be assured that these worries are needless; *the patient is not radioactive*.

Daily Activities

Many people go directly from treatment to their job, school, or home to engage in their usual activities. Others find that they are very tired following each treatment and need to go home to rest until the next one. As the cancer cells are destroyed, waste products build up in the blood, sapping energy from the rest of the body. You may be told to drink a few quarts of liquid each day to aid in the removal of these waste products. This will help to restore your usual energy level.

Special precautions. Your skin needs careful attention during the period of treatment. Skin should be very gently cleansed, and you should avoid rubbing, pressure, or irritation from tight clothes, scratchy or harsh fabrics on the treatment area. Also avoid deodorants, perfumes, colognes, certain cosmetics, and products containing alcohol. You shouldn't shave the area either (although your doctor may say it's all right to do so with an electric razor). Unless your physician approves, do not use tape or Band-Aids there, and avoid heat in the form of hot-water bottles, heating pads, sun lamps, and sunlight. Also avoid extreme cold or applying ice-packs to the area. Do not use ointments, salves, or cream except if ordered to. Substitute cotton for synthetic underclothing. You should discuss all of these issues with your doctor or nurse since skin care to the area being treated may vary. The nurse may give you special creams or lotions.

Sometimes the skin in the treatment area becomes very sensitive and will become flaky, itchy, red, or look tanned. This is a normal reaction, and although it should be called to the attention of the physician or nurse, it is not cause for alarm. Skin reactions may occur in the area where the radiation leaves the body, as well as where it enters.

Side Effects From External Radiation

Modern radiation techniques and machinery produce far less side effects than were experienced during the early years of radiotherapy. However, certain side effects are sometimes unavoidable. Chapter 11 discusses side effects in more detail.

Side effects are most likely to occur in those normal cells that are most radiosensitive. These cells, which have a rapid rate of cell division, include the cells of the bone marrow (red blood cells, white blood cells, and platelets), the gastrointestinal tract (mucous membranes of the mouth, esophagus, stomach, and intestines), the genitourinary tract (ureters and bladder), hair follicles, and gonads. When these sensitive cells are located within or closely adjacent to the area being radiated, they are at risk of being damaged, causing side effects.

Many precautions are taken to avoid or minimize these side effects. Lead blocks and shields are used to protect the normal body tissue in the area of the treatment field, and great care is taken to avoid damage to the reproductive organs and to any areas that might suffer from permanent damage. (Men who receive radiation to the reproductive areas may wish to consider banking sperm in a sperm bank. Discuss this with the physician prior to treatment.) It is important to note that not everyone who receives radiation experiences side effects.

During the period in which you are having radiation treatment, the physician may order X rays to determine if the tumor is shrinking. You may also undergo regular blood tests to be sure that the radiation is not lowering your white blood or platelet count too much. Based on this information, the radiotherapist may want you to take a few days off from treatment to allow your blood count to get closer to normal.

Other tests may also be ordered, especially if you are experiencing side effects.

When your treatment is completed, you will probably have one or more appointments with the radiotherapist, who will want to check on your response to the treatment. The radiotherapist will send a complete report to the referring physician (surgeon or medical oncologist), who will discuss it with you.

INTERNAL RADIATION

Internal radiation is a much newer technique than external radiation, but it is now an established therapy for certain cancers and is available in many communities as well as all major medical centers.

Internal radiation, as we discussed earlier, involves the direct placement of radioactive material into the body, either by temporary implantation or in the form of pills or injection. When radioactive material is placed close to the cancerous tissue, inside the body, it can concentrate radiation where it is needed and spare the surrounding tissues. These sources of radiation are usually contained in a device such as a needle, wire, seed, or capsule. The procedure must be done in the hospital. The radioactive implants may remain anywhere from one day to a week or two. Occasionally, implants remain in the body indefinitely but cease to become radioactive after a short, specified time.

When radiation is given by injection or pill, it is usually a "one-time" procedure.

Temporary radioactive implants. If your doctor decides on this therapy, you will have to spend some time in the hospital. In gynecological cancers, for instance, you are taken to the operating room, where the doctor inserts an applicator or container into your vagina. X rays determine if any adjustments are necessary, and gauze packing is often placed around the container to keep it in place. After you have returned to your room, the radioactive material, which is encased in plastic, is slid into the applicator already inside you. Such intracavitary implants are also performed for cancers in other body cavities and organs, such as those of the breast, head, and neck.

One type of implant, called *interstitial*, consists of needles made of radioactive material. These needles may be inserted directly into the small areas or spaces of an organ or tissue that is cancerous. These temporary implants are usually removed in the hospital room after three to fourteen days.

During the period in which you have the implant inside you, some radiation may be emitted from your body. For this reason you will be in a private room (at semiprivate rates), and while staff will administer to your needs, their visits will be brief. Visitors will be limited; children and pregnant or nursing women will not be able to visit you. Visitors should stay for only about forty-five minutes to one hour, and should remain six feet away from you.

If the radiation material is encased in a sealed source, neither your clothes, bed linens, nor body excretions will become radioactive, and as soon as the radioactive source is removed from your body, you will not, in any way, remain radioactive.

Your activities may be limited during therapy, in order to avoid dislodging the implant. Breast-implant patients can sometimes walk around the room, but many other patients will have to stay in bed.

You may experience fatigue, discomfort, or pain during this period. The physician or nurse should tell you what to expect. Medication will be ordered for pain or discomfort.

Permanent implants. Radioactive implants are sometimes left permanently in the prostate, tongue, or mouth, rather than being surgically removed. The implant does not remain radioactive; within a specified period (usually only a few days), radiation will no longer be emitted from your body. Those implants that remain do not cause pain or discomfort. Friends and family will be able to come as close to you as you wish with no fear of contamination. Men who have permanent implants in their prostate are able to have sexual intercourse with no risk to their partner. (Check with your physician when sexual activity may begin.)

Intravenous injection or pills. Radioactive material can be given orally or by injection, so that it mingles with body fluids and travels to the tumor and elsewhere. For instance, to treat thyroid glands, the patient swallows radioactive iodine. Radioactive material can also be injected into the bloodstream or directly into the tumor. This is a safe, highly effective method of treating certain cancers, and is most often done in a radiotherapist's office. It does not cause side effects or endanger healthy cells.

Intraoperative radiation. In a newer technique, still being developed at some large medical centers, a strong dose of radiation is aimed directly at the cancer in the operating room, following surgical removal of all or part of the tumor. Normal tissue is shielded and protected from the radiation. So far, results have been encouraging.

Cost of Radiotherapy

Radiotherapy is expensive, but in most instances insurance will pay for it. If you have private insurance, Medicare, or Medicaid, you are unlikely to incur substantial additional expenses. Discuss this with the radiotherapist and the patient-accounts department of the hospital where you are being treated. See also Chapter 15.

New techniques, new machinery, and more highly trained radiotherapists in more centers throughout the nation are delivering stronger and, paradoxically, more tolerable radiation treatments to cancer patients. Used instead of, before, or after surgery or chemotherapy, radiation therapy is yielding excellent results in many formerly resistant cancers.

Chapter 6
Chemotherapy

Chemotherapy is the treatment of cancer (or any disease) with combinations of different chemical substances or drugs that work internally and invisibly throughout the body.

Chemotherapy can be used to suppress cancer before, with, instead of, or after surgery or radiation to treat cancer. When given along with other treatments, it is often referred to as *adjuvant chemotherapy*. Chemotherapy can shrink tumors before they are surgically removed or treated with radiation. These drugs can also effectively remove or destroy the remnants of cancer that surgery and/or radiotherapy are unable to destroy. In addition, chemotherapy can ease and control pain and other symptoms of cancer.

Alone, or following nonradical surgery, chemotherapy can cure a number of cancers, such as some leukemias and lymphomas, testicular cancers and osteosarcomas. It can prolong survival and palliate many cancers that were once untreatable.

Not all cancers are treated with chemotherapy, but anytime cancer is suspected or confirmed, a patient should have a consultation with a medical oncologist, as described in Chapter 2. The oncologist will, in addition to general recommendations about treatment, evaluate the need for chemotherapy.

If you are going to have chemotherapy, it is this medical oncologist who will plan the treatment. Most likely you will go to his office, or the clinic where he works, for the treatments, but it is possible that the oncologist will confer with your own family physician in whose office you will get treatments.

In some offices or clinics, the actual administration of the drugs may be given to a physician's assistant or clinical-oncology nurse trained in these procedures. The physician carefully supervises all treatments.

How Chemotherapy Works

Chemotherapy actually kills cancer cells, which of course stops them from growing and reproducing. It can affect cells of any size:

those large enough to form tumors, and those so small that they cannot be seen even by today's newest, most sensitive diagnostic tests. Scientists know these unseen cells are there because even when a tumor is destroyed or removed, cancer sometimes recurs. By destroying all or most of these tiny colonies of cancer cells, which may have broken away from the primary tumor, recurrences can often be prevented or postponed. For this reason early and prompt treatment . . . just after diagnosis and surgery—rather than after a recurrence—can help to achieve long-term control or cure of cancer.

Is chemotherapy still "new" and experimental? Chemotherapy is certainly not new; it is based on some of the oldest known treatments for disease. For instance, primitive people used plant extracts to treat disease, and many of the most modern, sophisticated anticancer drugs *are* plant extracts. Although the term *chemotherapy* is usually associated with cancer, it also applies to treatment with drugs in general—treatment of such diseases as tuberculosis, bacterial infections, and syphilis.

It was in the years just following World War II that chemotherapy first began to be used effectively for the treatment of cancer. During the war, nitrogen mustard gas was found to have anticancer properties, and soon the search for more and better drugs was underway. Initially, only a few drugs were used, and they were administered one at a time. By 1960 there were seventeen anticancer drugs in use. The concept of combined chemotherapy was then introduced, which led the way for newer and more effective treatments. More recently, many extremely powerful new drugs have been introduced, and new combinations and new ways of using old drugs are yielding better results than was previously even imagined. Drugs may be combined during a single treatment session or administered on successive days or even spaced widely apart. Because cancer cells differ from normal cells, they multiply and spread indiscriminately, sometimes simultaneously or at different rates. Thus, doctors use a variety of drugs that act on different cell mechanisms and inhibit each of the various patterns of growth.

Despite the proven track record of chemotherapy for many cancers, some physicians still delay recommending it until patients have a recurrence of their disease. This has resulted in the mistaken notion among many people that chemotherapy was either experimental or reserved only for those patients who were extremely ill. Today, we know that *early* chemotherapy, like early diagnosis, is a most effective weapon against cancer.

Types of Drugs

There are five major types of drugs and over one hundred individual drugs used on cancer, and each works in its own way. It is now widely recognized that certain drugs in combination are far more effective than the same drugs given separately. It is almost impossible for a nonscientist to fully master or understand the detailed workings of the different anticancer agents, and curious as it may seem, even scientists don't always know exactly how each drug works. If that seems strange to you, you might be interested to know that even though aspirin has been around for more than eighty years, its precise mechanism still isn't fully understood.

Alkylating agents cause a direct chemical interaction with the cells, blocking their multiplication. They affect cancer cells in all phases of the life cycle, even if they are not dividing, by interfering with DNA and RNA in the cells' nuclei. Among these drugs are Cytoxan and Thio-TEPA and Cis-platinum (one of the newest and most powerful drugs). Cis-platinum is used to treat a variety of cancers, and it has had a profound success in curing and increasing survival for many patients.

Antimetabolites are described by scientists as "fraudulent nutrients" because they "fool" the cells into absorbing them. Once there, they interfere with further growth and the cancer cells' natural inclination to keep copying themselves. Methrotrexate and 5-Fluorouracil (5-FU) are examples of antimetabolites. Methrotrexate acts as an antagonist, competing with one of the B vitamins (folic acid), thereby inhibiting cancer-cell growth.

Patients taking antimetabolites are often told by their physician not to take excessive amounts of certain vitamins of the B group, particularly folic acid, since they can interfere with the antimetabolites' mission of starving the cancer cells.

Mitotic inhibitors work to prevent cancer cells from splitting (undergoing mitosis) and dividing normally, thus interfering with the process needed to produce more cells. Examples of mitotic inhibitors are Velban (vinblastine) and Oncovin (vincristine), both of which are derivatives of the periwinkle plant.

Tumoricidal antibiotics interfere with cell division and growth. They are made from natural substances such as soil fungi. Examples of these drugs are Adriamycin and Bleomycin.

Hormones occur naturally in the body, where they turn on or off growth or activity of certain cells in organs. As stated earlier, some cancers are dependent on natural male or female hormones for their growth, so when the opposite hormone (or antihormone) is used as treatment, the cancer growth is inhibited.

Both prostate cancer and some breast cancers are dependent upon male hormones for growth. In these instances, a synthetic female hormone, stilbesterol, is given to block the male hormones. Other breast cancers are dependent on female hormones for growth. In these instances Nolyadex (tamoxifin), an anti-estrogen, and androgens (male hormones) are given to block the female hormones.

Steroid compounds, which include such hormones as adrenal cortical compounds (related to cortisone), are used to combat several types of cancers. Some hormones are relatively nontoxic, but all can produce some undesirable side effects in certain circumstances.

The use of hormones in cancer treatment is sometimes referred to as *hormonotherapy* or *hormone therapy*. Hormone therapy is often administered instead of, prior to, or in addition to chemotherapy. In appendix V you will find a complete list of drugs used in chemotherapy.

As you can see, even from this brief overview of chemotherapy, the various drugs work in different ways to shrink tumors or to halt further cell growth and shrink tumors. Some are used alone, others in combination. Some act as catalysts to make other drugs more potent.

Although these drugs specifically attack cancer cells, they can also interfere to a limited extent with some functions of certain normal cells, causing some of the side effects that I'll discuss in more detail in Chapter 12.

ADMINISTRATION OF THE DRUGS

To reach the cancer cells and be effective, medication must enter the bloodstream. You may take pills orally (by mouth) in tablet or capsule form, after which they are absorbed through the lining of the stomach before entering the bloodstream. Alternatively, the drugs can be injected into a muscle (intramuscular, or IM, injection), eventually entering the bloodstream, or they can be injected directly into the bloodstream through a vein (intravenous, or IV, injection). Or they may be dripped slowly into a vein by means of gravity (IV infusion). These treatments are given in a doctor's office or at the outpatient clinic of a hospital. In some instances, and with some particular drugs, you may need to stay in the hospital for anywhere from one to several days.

Beginning chemotherapy. When you begin chemotherapy, your physician may choose to give you an induction dose—large amounts of the drug over the first few days—followed by smaller, maintenance doses on a daily or weekly basis. Sometimes, for certain drugs, doctors may want you to begin treatment in the hospital so that you can be very carefully monitored. After that you may be treated as an outpatient.

It is important to realize that the method and time sequence of your treatments may be unrelated to the state of your disease. Someone who enters the hospital monthly may be no sicker than someone who takes one small pill at home on a regular basis.

Chemotherapy pills are not always taken daily. Your doctor may prescribe them in cycles of a few days in a row, or during two weeks each month, or on any number of other schedules. Although this scheme may not make much sense to you, it has been planned that way for good reason. The medical oncologist has a thorough understanding of tumor cell biology and of pharmacology and knows how to design routes and schedules to ensure the optimum delivery of drugs to the tumor when it is in the phase most sensitive to the drugs.

Different drugs have different time sequences for their effectiveness, and since the drugs affect normal as well as cancerous cells, the drug-free intervals allow normal cells to repair themselves. The drugs can continue to work against the cancer cells during the intervals when you are not taking the medication, because the cancer cells do not repair themselves as fast as normal cells do. The doses and cycles planned by your doctor are based on many factors including your age and size, and whether the drugs are given singly or in combination.

You must follow the schedule exactly. It is very important that you trust that the specificity of this schedule is important and abide by it. Your physician also trusts that you follow it exactly, since he cannot stand over you at home and be sure you are taking your medication. Nor can he pull you into his office with a hook! It is amazing how many people skip appointments either because they "feel fine," or are too tired. Keep your appointments as scheduled, and *always* phone your oncologist if you notice any side effects or other problems.

It may be helpful to hang a large wall calendar in the room where you will be taking the pills and to mark it accordingly. A large X on the dates when you should take your pills will serve as a good reminder. If you are taking different pills and the schedule is more complicated, you may find it helpful to make the X's with a different color for each type of pill and put a color key at the bottom of the calendar. You might also note the time of day you are supposed to take the medication, and check off the time *after* you take the pill. It's easy to forget you have taken a pill; making check marks will avoid frantic counting of remaining pills to know exactly what you have done.

Comparing notes. You will probably meet many other people undergoing chemotherapy. Coworkers, friends, relatives, friends of friends, as well as patients in the waiting room or in cancer-support groups, may want to "compare notes" with you. It is helpful to give each other tips on coping with chemotherapy and the cancer experience, and to share your feelings and fears, but it is *not* helpful to compare treatment plans. Your schedule was prepared especially for *you*, and someone else's was prepared for *him*, and it is unlikely that your needs are exactly the same.

Delivery systems. In addition to the traditional methods of giving medications (orally, by injections, etc.), new "delivery systems" have been developed that allow drugs and other substances to be administered to the body.

For instance, drugs are sometimes injected directly into a tumor by means of a catheter. This treatment is called *regional perfusion*, and it is designed to destroy cancer tissue with minimal damage to normal surrounding tissue.

Drugs can also be introduced directly into the circulatory system, avoiding repeated intramuscular and intravenous injections.

One of the delivery systems that many physicians, nurses, and patients find especially effective is the right-atrial catheter, sometimes referred to as the Broviac-Hickman catheter. Once it is inserted, patients are able to avoid repeated injections and "sticks" for blood samples and treatments. This catheter, or tube, provides a pathway for medications and nutrients, and also permits blood samples to be taken for tests. It is usually inserted (entrance site) into the upper chest, resting on the right atrium of the heart, and comes out (exit site) through the chest wall a few inches below the entrance site.

Insertion of the catheter takes about an hour and is performed in an inpatient or outpatient operating room. The surgeon will give you a local anesthetic to numb the area, and he will use a fluoroscope to guide him in placing the catheter in the proper location. It is a fairly minor procedure, and many patients are up and on their way right after it is done.

You will have stitches in both entrance and exit sites; these stitches will be removed in about a week or ten days. Continual care of the exit site and of the catheter itself is necessary, but you and perhaps a designated family member will be taught how to do this. You will have to flush the catheter out three or four times a week with an anticoagulant (medication used to prevent blood from clotting), such as Heparin, to prevent dried blood and other particles from blocking the catheter.

A more normal life is possible than with other therapies, according to some patients, who explain that after insertion of the catheter they no longer have to worry about frequent injections, or about the pain and swelling that sometimes occurs following repeated injections and blood tests. The catheter does not interfere with their usual activities.

Once the incisions have healed, you can shower and even swim (with extra careful attention after you come out of the water). You can play tennis and golf, dance, drive a car, and engage in sexual activity. You may *prefer* not to wear low necklines, but generally, you will be able to wear most of the same clothes you have always worn. You certainly can wear a bathing suit. When people inquired about the tube coming out of his chest, one handsome bachelor liked to tell everyone at his pool club that he had decided to provide a direct route to his heart, making it easier for all the lovely young women who were sunning themselves to capture his attention.

Some patients keep the catheter in place for up to two years, or through the entire course of chemotherapy. The catheter can be easily and quickly removed in a physician's office.

Most people make use of the catheter only in their doctor's office or in the hospital, but some patients are able to give themselves medication or nutritional supplements through it while they are at home.

Implantable pump. An even more direct method for delivery of drugs, available in a number of medical centers, involves the implantation of a pump inside the patient that releases the prescribed quantity of chemicals directly into the site of disease. The pump is about the size of a hockey puck and usually consists of a hermetically sealed reservoir, a precise pumping mechanism, and a self-contained energy source, all linked to the drug delivery site via a soft catheter. It can mete out a minute flow of chemotherapy or pain medication, usually at a constant rate. Because drugs can be delivered directly to the site of the disease, dosages can be increased to a rate far greater than is possible through conventional intravenous methods. This avoids many of the side effects on normal tissue that would otherwise occur. The pump, which is also available as an external unit, enables patients to continue therapy at home rather than being hospitalized. It has been especially useful in treating cancer of the liver.

Measuring the Effectiveness of the Drugs

Your doctor has many ways of knowing if the chemotherapy is effectively destroying your cancer cells. He examines you physically for signs of tumor regression, orders X rays, scans, and many blood and urine laboratory tests at regular intervals.

You yourself cannot truly determine how you are doing. Naturally, if you feel any growths or recognize some changes (see Appendix II), you must promptly report them to your doctor; do not wait until your next appointment. But it is generally difficult for the patient and his family to know whether the chemotherapy is doing its intended job.

There is *no* relationship between side effects from chemotherapy and the effectiveness of the drugs in controlling cancer.

Testing New Drugs

New drugs are always tested extensively in laboratories long before they are given to humans. They are tested in test-tube cultures of cancer cells (in vitro) or on animals (in vivo) and must prove to have a wide range of safety and be effective against animal cancers *before* they are given to cancer patients.

The initial study of new drugs on patients is called Phase I testing. It usually involves fifty to two hundred patients who have advanced disease and on whom doctors have used all accepted forms of treatment. Even so, these new drugs are used carefully.

Phase II testing includes drugs that have gone through earlier human testing but are still being carefully investigated to determine the extent of their effectiveness and to determine the best dosage schedules. These drugs are usually available only through physicians who obtain them directly or indirectly through the National Cancer Institute. However, those physicians who are not directly involved in a study will sometimes work in cooperation with a doctor who is doing Phase II drug testing, or they can send a patient to this doctor.

New drugs are not necessarily the most effective, but new combinations and new and constant improvements in dosage and timing schedules can result in improved patient response.

Only 2 percent of patients receive Phase I or Phase II drugs. The vast majority receive Phase III drugs. These are the drugs that have been thoroughly tested and investigated on a very large scale and are approved for use, but may still be undergoing study for further information on optimum doses or combinations. Many physicians prescribe these drugs as standard chemotherapy.

If you are getting a Phase I or Phase II drug that is still under investigation or evaluation, it may be available only under certain requirements. Thus you may have to agree to take the drug in a hospital or clinic setting where special record-keeping can be done. You will also have to sign an "informed consent" agreement. This agreement explains procedures, discomforts, risks, benefits, and possible alternative methods of managing the disease. It also explains that you can withdraw anytime, without loss of medical attention and care.

Other patients with similar cancers in other cities may be undergoing the same careful observation and reporting, as part of a cooperative study. They may all be receiving the same *protocol*, a predetermined treatment plan for groups of patients.

Just because you are getting new drugs or new schedules does not mean that your disease is so advanced that they are "trying anything."

Instead, it may mean that you are receiving the most current cancer management treatment available, one that will increase your chances for cure or long-term control of your disease.

ACTIVITIES WHILE RECEIVING CHEMOTHERAPY

Most patients who are receiving chemotherapy are able to carry on their usual activities, at least most of the time. Some people find that for a few days after certain treatments they have to take it easy. However, those patients who have jobs, or take care of their families or households, find that they can resume most of their responsibilities, even though they may require more rest or some "days off." You may wish to ask your doctor or clinic to consider your personal needs regarding appointments. If you work, you may prefer to have an injection late in the day, or even on a Friday, so you can use the following hours or days to relax before going back to work. If you are a parent, you may prefer to have the injections on a weekday, while your children are in school or when baby-sitters are available, to be free to enjoy a pleasant family weekend.

Some people cope best by taking it "one day at a time"; others need goals or plans for the future. There is no denying that it is complicated and discouraging to arrange your life around the treatment schedule; it serves as a constant reminder of your disease.

For many people, one of the most difficult things about undergoing chemotherapy is the feeling that the schedule is taking over their lives. Knowing that others feel the same way, and learning from each other about little ways that still give you a sense of control, can be very helpful. Always try to remember that the chemotherapy is working to control your cancer. But, as one patient said, "It's still a bummer." If the chemotherapy is really getting you down, consider counseling, or join a support or self-help group.

Side Effects

Some people have no side effects; others have many. Most have just some, and then only at times.

Like radiation, chemotherapy may destroy some normal cells as well as cancer cells. Unlike radiation, which just reaches targeted locations and some adjacent areas, most kinds of chemotherapy reach all areas of the body. Thus, side effects are more likely to be experienced from chemotherapy than from radiation. In addition, chemotherapy may be spread out over a period of months, rather than just weeks, so side effects may seem to be eternal. But they *will* stop.

The normal cells that are most likely to be affected by chemotherapy are those of the upper gastrointestinal tract, the bone marrow, hair follicles, and skin. The drugs can also affect muscles and nerves and sometimes cause changes in certain sexual characteristics.

Most of the side effects are temporary, and just as all patients are somewhat unique in their particular disease and response to treatment, so they are unique in their individual tolerance to the drugs. For instance, one patient may become so nauseated that he needs strong antinausea medication when he receives a particular drug, but you may go straight from the doctor's office to a favorite restaurant. Or the drug that makes you nauseous during one cycle may have no effect the next time around.

Again, let me repeat one important point that a patient who is receiving chemotherapy must understand: *There is no relationship between side effects and drug effectiveness.* Thus, if there are no side effects, it does not mean the drug isn't working. And severe side effects do not necessarily mean that the drug is working effectively.

Most patients believe that the benefits of chemotherapy far outweigh the inconveniences—occasional sick days or even several miserable days in a row. Those patients for whom chemotherapy (because of the particular drug, frequency, or individual reactions) is really horrendous often find it difficult to believe that the treatment is worthwhile. It is difficult for them to feel they are getting better when they are feeling so sick. They are tempted to refuse more treatment. But once the therapy is completed, they have returned to normal activities, and their disease is under control or even cured (as in testicular cancer), they will encourage newly diagnosed patients to go through it. And over and over, these patients *do* accept treatment again if they have a recurrence. Some of these patients are discovering, and it is important to note, that *new antinausea drugs can prevent much of the intense nausea that so many patients experienced as side effects a few years ago.*

Since side effects vary from drug to drug and from patient to patient, neither your doctor nor this book can give you an exact prediction of how *you* will react. In Chapter 12 I will discuss in more detail the kinds of side effects that can occur from chemotherapy, and the ways in which to minimize, reduce, alleviate, and sometimes even prevent them.

Other medications can interfere with chemotherapy, so before you continue with or take any new medications, discuss them with your doctor. Even those drugs that you consider harmless such as aspirin, antacids, and vitamin supplements, may occasionally interfere with some chemotherapy drugs. Before you begin chemotherapy, give the doctor a list of any medications (and that includes vitamins!) that you take regularly or occasionally. If you aren't sure of the exact name of the drug or the dosage, bring the bottles with you on your first visit.

Don't take any *other* drugs (even those you can buy at the drugstore without a prescription) without first consulting your doctor. If, for some reason, you have occasion to see another doctor, such as an eye doctor or dentist, be sure to tell him that you are receiving chemotherapy, and give this doctor a list of the specific drugs.

In Appendix III you will find a list of medications that should not be taken without approval from your medical oncologist. You should keep a list of any and all medications you currently take. Many pharmacies today have your entire "drug profile" (any prescription drugs you ordered there) on their computer, so your pharmacist may be able to help fill in any of your memory gaps.

Drinking alcohol. Most patients can enjoy and tolerate occasional wine, beer, mixed drinks, or cocktails. There are some circumstances in which alcohol may have to be restricted or avoided. Be sure to ask your physician whether you need to limit or omit alcohol consumption.

Does chemotherapy lose its effect after a while? This can happen. But if it does, your doctor will put you on another drug or combination of drugs. There is more than one effective drug or drug combination for almost every form of cancer, and switching to a new combination is often prescribed deliberately just as a precaution against tumor resistance and recurrence of disease.

Remember that new drugs are constantly being developed and old drugs are being improved; chemotherapy is a steadily improving means of treating cancer.

Will I always need to have chemotherapy? Some people remain on small doses of mild drugs long after there is no evidence of disease. Other patients remain on chemotherapy for a fixed period of time; perhaps one, two, or three years. The decision is based on statistical and scientific information on your type of cancer and is planned to give you the optimum treatment for your disease.

If your adverse reaction to the drugs is too violent, to the point of toxicity (where side effects became serious or potentially dangerous), your doctor may interrupt treatment for certain periods of time. This allows him to judge your response and plan future treatments to the best possible advantage.

Cost of Chemotherapy

Undergoing chemotherapy can be expensive. Aside from the physician's fees, there are the high costs of some drugs and the many laboratory tests and X rays necessary to monitor your progress. Basic medical insurance does not always cover all these costs, but Medicare and many major-medical policies may cover anywhere from 80 to 100 percent of them. Discuss your financial situation and insurance coverage with your doctor or his office manager.

Many patients choose to get their treatment at major teaching hospitals, in a clinic setting where the care is excellent and attentive. These institutions will often accept whatever insurance you have, or may adjust fees to meet your personal financial situation.

If you are not able to work, you may be able to get disability insurance from your place of employment, and you should apply for government disability. Medicare is available for those people under sixty-five who are disabled.

If your expenses are great and your income is dwindling, you may be eligible for Medicaid or some other government-assisted medical insurance. The social work or patients account department at your hospital may be able to give you information and advice on obtaining this kind of aid. See Chapter 15 for further information on insurance and other financial concerns.

No person need go without chemotherapy because of the cost involved. Somewhere, in your own community, help will be available. The American Cancer Society or your local department of social services will be able to advise you on the best way to afford treatment if you are unable to find help through your physician or hospital.

Chapter 7

Immunotherapy and Other Promising Treatments

Although surgery, radiation, and chemotherapy remain the chief methods of treating and curing cancer, a number of new treatments are being used, mainly in conjunction with traditional treatments.

IMMUNOTHERAPY

Immunotherapy is the attempt to stimulate and strengthen the body's own natural defenses for protection against and recovery from disease. This treatment is still fairly new, but it shows promise of being effective against some cancers, especially when used in combination with chemotherapy.

Understanding the body's immune system helps to understand the potential of immunotherapy. The body has an amazing ability to recognize and destroy foreign invaders before they endanger our health. Without this ability, even the slightest cut, infection, or minor illness could be fatal. The body recognizes these foreign invaders, which are called antigens, and reacts to them in several different ways. White blood cells attack bacteria and stimulate the production of antibodies in the blood plasma. These antibodies circulate through the bloodstream and attack the antigens. What's more, the antibodies continue to circulate, recognizing the same invaders if they try to reenter the body. This explains why certain (but not all) childhood illnesses give us lifelong immunity. It also explains the principle of vaccination, the use of weak antigens to stimulate antibody production. This "fools" the body into thinking you have the disease, and since it's in a weak form, your antibodies can combat it easily, while learning to recognize those antigens and be on guard for future attacks of the disease.

There are three major forms of immunological activity:

The *antibody response* is produced by B cells, which are manufactured in the bone marrow. These cells produce the antibodies that help defend the body against infection or toxic substances.

The *cellular immune response* is produced by lymphocytes (or T cells), which mature in the thymus gland and are stimulated by antigens to circulate through the body.

Natural killer (NK) cells are stimulated by viral infections, possibly through production of interferon, a chemical substance that also is naturally released by the body in response to viral infections. This natural resistance differs from the immunity acquired by previous exposure and is not caused by B or T cells.

It is now widely recognized that individuals with a suppressed or deficient immune system are vulnerable and prone to many diseases, including cancer. It is also recognized that cancer patients are vulnerable to infections and other illnesses, because their immunity is low.

It has *not* been proved that a suppressed immune system will necessarily lead to cancer, or that everyone who develops cancer had a suppressed or deficient immune system before developing cancer. Current studies are attempting to determine if the reason most people *don't* get cancer is because their immune system (particularly the NK-cell system) is thriving.

Stress appears to weaken the immune system; some studies have demonstrated that environmental, emotional, or physical stress may precede the diagnosis of cancer. This gives credence to the theory that a poor immune system allows the cancer cells to develop and overpower healthy cells.

There have been a very small number of documented cases in which cancer has spontaneously disappeared in patients, never to appear again. In some other patients, tumors have spontaneously shrunk or disappeared only to reappear at a later date. The immune system may be responsible for these phenomena. Tumors have also sometimes shrunk following severe infections or high fevers. All these findings have led scientists to seek more definitive answers to the relationship between cancer and the immune system.

Why doesn't the body form antibodies to fight cancer cells as it does to fight bacteria? There are many theories: One is that cancer cells are capable of eluding the immune system; another is that because cancer cells have developed from the body's own normal cells, the immune system doesn't perceive them as foreign invaders.

Theoretically, improving and repairing the immune system of cancer patients should lead to greater control and even cure of the disease, *if* cancer is the result of a suppressed immune system. This theory, however, must be studied much more thoroughly before it can be put to practical use.

Researchers are developing and testing various vaccines and other products that are intended to "help the body help itself" by persuading the immune system to recognize and reject cancer cells. At this time, immunological methods alone have not been able to provide any predictable control of any of the diverse forms of cancer. But after most of a tumor has been destroyed by surgery, radiation, or chemotherapy, this approach has shown some promise as an adjunct, helping to eliminate the last remnants of active cancer cells in the body.

Immunotherapy used with chemotherapy is sometimes referred to as *chemoimmunotherapy*.

Nonspecific Immunotherapy

The chemicals used in immunotherapy can be injected systemically to the entire body by an injection under the skin or into a vein. They can also be injected directly into the tumor or taken by mouth. Nonspecific immunotherapy is intended to mobilize the immune response in a general way, so that the white blood cells will recognize the cancerous cells as foreign invaders and attack them. Immunotherapy may induce a very low-grade infection much like that which occurs after a person receives a vaccine against such diseases as rubella and smallpox.

One of the more common types of immunotherapy is called BCG (bacillus Calmette-Guerin), which is a mixture of live organisms. Though it was initially developed as a vaccine against tuberculosis, many oncologists now give it to their cancer patients who are receiving chemotherapy.

Another type of immunotherapy is MER (methanol extracted residue), which is extracted from BCG and made from killed organisms.

Immunotherapy may produce some side effects, such as tiredness, fever, inflammation or mild pain around the site of the treatment. Occasionally, chills or swelling of lymph nodes may occur.

Interferon. In 1957 two scientists in London discovered that influenza-infected chick embryo cells released a substance that, when added to *other* cells, made *those* cells resistant to viruses. The substance, named *interferon* for its ability to "interfere" with virus infections, is released naturally by animals and humans as a response to invading viruses.

Interferon recognizes, suppresses, and/or destroys the tumor cells.

It can also stimulate the NK cells and T cells, triggering the immune system. In high doses it can also *suppress* certain components of the immune system, so it must be used with considerable caution.

When the potential of interferon was first announced, only the natural substance was available—and in very short supply, since only human interferon could be used for humans. Since then it has been synthesized, and a great deal of money and time has gone into the scientific study of its effects upon cancer patients.

But interferon has not lived up to its early hyped-up media promise. While it has shown dramatic success in the treatment of an unusual cancer called hairy-cell leukemia, and is useful in treating multiple myeloma, it only slows the rate of growth and division of cells in many other cancers. In still others, it is completely ineffective.

Interferon alone does not at this time replace any conventional treatments for such common cancers as those of breast or lung. It appears to work best in combination with chemotherapy, and in the future it will probably have an important role as an adjunct to surgery and radiation therapy as well.

Tumor-specific antigens. In this form of immunotherapy, cancer cells from the patient are collected and grown in a laboratory culture, then treated with various chemicals that uncover the antigens. These treated cancer cells are injected back into the patient in the hope that, like a vaccination, they will produce an immune response to the tumor in the patient.

Bone-Marrow Transplants

Leukemias and lymphomas can be treated effectively with bone-marrow transplants. Those patients who have received a great deal of radiation and chemotherapy, and whose bone marrow is still diseased, may profit from the transplant of healthy, compatible bone marrow. Generally, the bone marrow is transplanted from a close relative.

The transplant involves a somewhat complex procedure in which the donor-recipient match is tested over a period of time. Then the donor is taken to an operating room, where the marrow is removed in much the same way as for a bone-marrow test (described in Chapter 3) but through several punctures, mainly in the hipbone. The donor may be anesthetized for this procedure.

The compatibility of bone-marrow blood types is more specific than in simple blood transfusions, and precision is essential to avoid a serious, life-threatening immune reaction in the recipient. For this reason the donor is usually a brother or sister of the patient. One young man said it was the finest gift he ever gave his brother.

Bone marrow can also be removed from patients who are in remission and stored until such time as they need it.

Hyperthermia

Hyperthermia, or heat therapy, is certainly not new as a treatment for cancer; it has been tried from time to time for thousands of years. There is no widely accepted explanation for the mechanism of the process, although many theories have been proposed. Despite its long history, it is still experimental, and although there have been some impressive results, it poses a potential risk to patients.

By raising overall body temperature to anywhere from 104 to 107 degrees F., doctors hope that a tumor will either go into spontaneous remission or become small enough to respond more readily to chemotherapy or radiation.

Hyperthermia is administered in several ways. In a rarely used technique of total-body hyperthermia, doctors raise the patient's body temperature by means of space-program technology. The patient is wrapped in plastic and placed under a hot-water blanket. Anything that enters the patient, such as intravenous fluids, is also heated. Other forms of hyperthermia include localized radiofrequency to the tumor, hyperthermia perfusion (in which blood in a specific area is heated), ultrasound, and microwave. Some of these treatments are combined with radiation, chemotherapy or surgery. Generally, the treatment periods are brief and given in a series over a few weeks. Hyperthermia has reduced some tumors sufficiently to permit surgery, or to slow the growth of recurrent tumors.

ON THE HORIZON

Researchers at National Cancer Institute and at medical institutions throughout the world continue to screen thousands of chemical compounds and extracts, and to practice new therapies, all in the hope of discovering more and better treatments for cancer.

Research takes time, and the development of a single drug from discovery to introduction is a long, expensive process requiring enormous funds, dedicated and innovative researchers, sophisticated facilities, and, after laboratory testing, special patient-care centers. Governments provide much of the funding, but private sources must also meet the challenge. Many legitimate not-for-profit fund-raising organizations and pharmaceutical companies contribute money to basic research and to programs at major medical institutions.

Regional cancer centers in the United States and abroad have formed cooperative oncology groups that pool data on the treatment of many patients with specific cancers, to ease the trials of new drugs and therapies. Because of this shared data, you can get the advantages of new drug treatment even if you do not live near a major research institute.

Investigations and studies of new treatments are always in progress, some of which are available in selected centers, and only to patients who meet very specific criteria. Many of these treatments are very promising; some have already proved effective for certain types of cancers in certain individuals. Others prove disappointing in the long run and are discarded as feasible therapies.

Transfer factor. This technique involves a protein substance obtained from the collection of white blood cells from a donor who has been tested to show specific immunity against the patient's own tumor. The white cells are removed from the blood of the donor and then injected into the patient, in the hope of increasing the patient's own immunity against the tumor. This type of immunotherapy is also called *adoptive therapy*. In a similar procedure, the patient's lymphocytes are removed from his blood and incubated with a natural substance called interleuken-2. This is then injected into the patient with additional interleuken-2. Such techniques have been effective in treating some noncancerous infections and are promising, but still experimental, as a cancer therapy.

Monoclonal antibodies are pure preparations of defensive immune-system compounds extracted from human or animal blood cells. They are currently used for diagnostic purposes, because of their ability to seek out and lock onto disease organisms. They have exciting potential for the future treatment of various kinds of cancer.

In a very high-tech process, a mouse is injected with antigens or live tumor cells from a human being. The mouse, in turn, produces antibodies against the injected material. Then the mouse's spleen is removed, and the cells that produced the antibodies are taken from the spleen and fused together with cancerous cells from another mouse. These cells, referred to as hybridomas, can then be cloned (replicated).

When these monoclonal antibodies are injected into a cancer patient, they seek out and attach themselves to specific proteins, such as those on the surface of cancer cells. The monoclonal antibodies can either attack the cancer cells or act like carriers, transporting strong chemotherapy substances or radioactive isotopes directly to them without damaging normal cells or causing side effects.

Although this technique is still highly experimental, a positive response has been reported in the treatment of some cancer patients. In many instances, however, the cancer cells seem to change themselves to such an extent that the monoclonal antibodies are "fooled" into no longer recognizing them.

Differentiation modifiers. These new anticancer drugs, also known as differentiation inducers, work to change cancer cells from their uncontrolled growth to more normal cell behavior *without* affecting normal cells. They are being tested on animals and may be ready for extensive testing in humans before very long.

The underlying concept is this: Cancerous cells began their life as normal cells but received faulty genetic information. Thus, they didn't "know" how to differentiate—that is, to develop into cells with clear-cut bodily functions, and then, at the right time, to stop proliferating. The differentiation modifiers would "tell" the cancerous cells to stop proliferating, reverse their abnormal course, and resume their normal characteristics.

The hope is that these differentiation modifiers may work well with conventional treatment in lowering the number of cancer cells so that complete destruction of the cancer is possible by other conventional methods.

Plasmapheresis. Transfusions of fresh blood plasma have resulted in partial tumor regression in some patients. The process requires plasma to be removed from a donor and transfused into the patient. White blood cells are removed from the patient, "washed," and returned to the bloodstream. The procedure is based on the concept that the patient's own plasma may contain some "blocking factors" that suppress the immune system.

Genetic Engineering. The entire potential of genetic engineering is exciting, but still on the horizon. Much of what we have discussed in the way of altering the immune system and changing cells from cancerous to normal comes within the realm of genetic engineering.

No Magic Bullet

A number of other treatments are being used experimentally, many still in test tubes and on animals, a few on humans. Immunotherapy shows promise, and other treatments are encouraging, but in 1986 the treatment of cancer is mostly dependent on the destruction of cancer cells by surgery, radiation, or chemotherapy.

There is no magic bullet for cancer—and probably never will be, because cancer is not one but many diseases. But there exists today an entire arsenal of weapons against cancer, affording patients far longer survival than was ever thought possible a generation ago. Many of these treatments can help you in your own fight against cancer.

Chapter 8
Unproven Cancer Treatments

Almost every patient has well-meaning relatives and friends who repeat stories from the media about foods, vitamins, drugs, and psychological therapies that have "cured" cancer. They may encourage you to try some of them.

Usually these stories are fictionalized, sensational, undocumented, inaccurate, and incomplete. Such therapies are unsupported by professionally published, detailed case studies available for review by medical scientists in recognized medical centers and impartial research organizations. Invariably, it has proved impossible for any scientific investigators in the field of cancer research to obtain results similar to those claimed in these stories. Often, the proponents of the "curative" drug or method will not even reveal the composition of the drug or give a precise description of how treatment is administered.

Patients have written books about their experiences with some of these unproven cures; such "true-life" stories can be very convincing. However, in many instances the patient never even had a confirmed (by biopsy) diagnosis of cancer. Other times they have received conventional treatment *prior* to the claimed "cure" and their remission can be attributed to the earlier treatment, to a temporary remission, or even to one of the rare natural remissions that cannot be attributed to any specific treatment.

No "miracle" drug has ever been scientifically demonstrated to cure cancer; in fact, no single substance, whether of proven usefulness or not, has even been able to reliably or consistently control or cure a wide range of cancers.

There are people who believe that good nutrition and vitamins *alone* can cure cancer. Good nutrition and vitamins *can* play a helpful role in your treatment plan, but only as an adjunct to more specific treatments. Your oncologist may indeed prescribe certain vitamins and/

or food supplements as part of your regular treatment plan. See Chapter 14 for more information about nutrition.

Why Do Patients Seek Unproven Cures?

Some people begin to explore the unproven cures almost as soon as they receive a diagnosis of cancer. They may know of people who weren't cured by conventional methods, and they wish to avoid the same fate. They may be fearful of treatments, having heard that "the side effects can be as bad as the disease." Their doctor's honesty about risks and the chances of a cure is discouraging when compared to the promises of a quack. The cost of cancer treatment also frightens many people, although it is usually available at an affordable price for anyone in their own community.

So the newly diagnosed patient may find the unproven methods very appealing. Products described as "natural" plants and vitamins promise to correct the body's "imbalance," which is named as the cause of the cancer. Sometimes a special diet purports to starve the cancer cells. These vigorous diets often end up starving the patients as well, robbing him of needed strength. Ironically, these "natural" products are often laced with toxic materials. Excess vitamin A, vitamin D, and selenium, for instance, are poisonous. Many of the "anticancer" vitamins aren't really vitamins and are not offered by any reputable pharmaceutical firm.

At a time of recurrence or when a recognized standard treatment does not seem to be making progress, patients may find it helpful to seek second or third opinions from conventional doctors who will, in all likelihood, recommend that they continue the same or similar treatment. When a patient becomes depressed or overcome by hopelessness, he will become particularly vulnerable to anyone or anything that holds out new hope. Sometimes representatives of those who offer the treatments even seek out patients and families in the waiting rooms of hospitals.

The printed media also have a great impact. Everything from sleazy, poorly printed pamphlets to well-printed hardcover books advocate some of these methods. Frequently the publication purports to give the "total" picture, but an impartial reader can easily see how skewed the material is on the side of the treatments being promoted.

Radio and television are highly persuasive as well. A glowing, healthy-looking patient is far more effective in "selling" an unproven treatment than the responsible articles condemning it are in convincing the public to avoid it.

Some so-called health organizations advertise meetings and open-to-the-public symposiums at which they describe their new treatments.

They often condemn the medical establishment as being too slow, uncaring, and greedy for money. Their meetings are emotionally charged and very potent. But nowhere is honest scientific data offered. It is always "about to be published," "awaiting further work"; or you'll hear, "We're too busy curing people to take time for formal publication of our data." Some detailed case reports indicate that after a patient was given chemotherapy or radiotherapy, the unproven method was then used. The improvement or cure of the patient was then ascribed to the last "treatment" rather than to the known benefit of standard therapy.

But still, it is easy to see why desperate or chronically discouraged patients are ready to try "anything." Unfortunately, many give up on conventional medicine when it still has a great deal to offer them. Such patients are not always ignorant. Many highly educated, sophisticated people have sought these unproven approaches. There is sometimes an element of truth behind the charges about the resistance of the medical establishment to new ideas. New understanding of the mind-body relationships, of the preventive and curative potential of activities such as fitness, sound nutrition, and stress reduction do lend an air of legitimacy to otherwise ineffective therapies.

Some of the treatments discussed in this chapter are simply unproved. Others are clearly ineffective, and still others have actually been demonstrated as harmful. *All* these treatments could prove fatal if patients stop or delay receiving recognized effective medical treatment.

Recognizing the Proponents of These "Cures"

It can be difficult to recognize the people who advocate these unprofessional treatments. Some are highly educated scientists who hold Ph.D.'s or even M.D.'s. Others may have a Ph.D. from a mail-order university, or their degree may be in something unrelated to medicine, or they list several unfamiliar degrees.

Some are charming, charismatic, or flamboyant people. Others have a low-key but earnest manner. Whatever their approach, they usually:

- are not associated with any established teaching hospital or university.
- have not had their work published in any reputable, scientific journal. (Your librarian can help advise you which journals are considered reputable.)
- claim that their work is *too* innovative; they don't want to waste valuable time fighting the establishment's rigid dogmatic beliefs.
- claim that organized medicine has a vested interest in postponing a cure for cancer.

- are unable to produce complete records of patients.
- are unwilling to consult with your own physician.
- refuse to divulge full information about the methods of treatment, or the "ingredients" in the substances they offer.
- have their own ways of diagnosing cancer and are not interested in other biopsy reports—often saying they are worthless, or that biopsies spread the cancer.
- produce letters and testimonials from many people, including writers, lawyers, statesmen, show-business personalities, and other well-meaning but scientifically untrained people. Sometimes they present endorsements from scientists, but never from anyone who is trained and experienced in the treatment of cancer.

Various Nostrums: Natural and Otherwise

For more than thirty years, a quack remedy called Laetrile enjoyed an undeserved popularity with cancer patients, although the medical establishment consistently scoffed at it and tried to persuade the public it was useless. Because it was illegal in the United States, Americans often spent their life savings to travel to Mexico and enter a clinic that dispensed Laetrile, which is formed from a substance found in apricot pits. Thousands of patients tried it. Medical opinion was unanimous in its opposition, the Food and Drug Administration banned it, but the public favored legalization. For years, legislators were beseeched to pass laws allowing Laetrile into the United States, and twenty-seven state legislatures actually did so.

The National Cancer Institute initially refused to do a study of Laetrile, because the drug showed no benefit when tried on animals or in other laboratory experiments. It seemed unethical to administer an almost certainly useless drug to cancer patients when drugs that had been proved useful were available. But public pressure persisted, and the NCI agreed to do a full-scale study.

The NCI study tested the drug in exactly the way those who offered Laetrile in the clinics recommended: It was administered in high doses and with a special diet. The result was no surprise to the researchers, who concluded:

- Laetrile is a toxic drug that is not effective as a cancer treatment. It offers no benefit to patients with advanced cancer.
- In addition, it is a cyanide-laden remedy, dangerously toxic at the recommended level.

A highly publicized case was that of a young boy who was receiving conventional treatment—with curative potential—at a hospital near his home in Massachusetts. His parents, no doubt well-meaning, but sadly misguided, chose to ignore medical advice and discontinued his chemotherapy. They took him to Mexico, where he received Laetrile. He died, the victim of an unproven treatment that amounted to nothing, as well as of the poisonous effects of the drug itself.

Years before the introduction of Laetrile, a drug named Krebiozen achieved fame in the cancer "underground." Like Laetrile, it appealed to the desperate. It, too, was proved worthless.

We certainly haven't seen the end of several highly promoted, totally worthless "wonder drugs."

Machines and Devices

Machines and other devices that are said to diagnose as well as treat cancer have been offered by nonprofessionals for many years. Some of them look harmless—and many probably *are*, but for the fact that the patient is not getting other, helpful treatment. Many of these machines look impressively like familiar conventional diagnostic tools, but unless they are approved by the FDA as safe *and* effective, or presently under study at a major teaching hospital or some other reputable institution, you can be fairly certain they are useless.

Vitamins

Some precancerous skin conditions can be combatted with vitamin A in safe, modest doses. But no vitamins will cure cancer. Cancer does not develop from a hidden vitamin deficiency. Neither vitamin C nor mega-vitamins or any others will cure or check cancer. Overdosing on vitamins can lead to toxicity. As I said earlier, vitamins are often prescribed or recommended by oncologists or surgeons as an adjunct to conventional treatment. Good nutritional intake, which includes vitamins, is helpful during treatment, and has a place in helping to prevent cancer, but in no way does it constitute a therapy in and of itself.

Fad Diets

There have been many fad diets suggested over the years that were purported to cure cancer. None of them has worked.

And now yet another diet is being promoted—and major bookstores as well as health-food stores sell literature describing it. It is called the macrobiotic diet. Several variations are recommended, not all of which provide adequate nutrition. The "ideal" macrobiotic diet is very restrictive, consisting entirely of grains. The macrobiotic diet recommended for cancer patients consists of 50 to 60 percent whole-grain cereals, 20 to 25 percent vegetables, 5 to 10 percent beans and sea vegetables, and 5 percent soups. Patients are advised to drink liquids only when they are thirsty, and they are told to chew each bite of food at least one hundred and preferably two hundred times. They are not supposed to eat any food within three hours of bedtime.

Most of the macrobiotic proponents believe that your thinking, behavior, and life-style are basic to the development of cancer. They make general and specific recommendations for altering your life-style as well as your diet. Many proponents view all traditional treatments for cancer—such as surgery, radiation, and chemotherapy—as "violent or artificial" and "toxic and unnatural." They will tell a cancer patient that his recovery has been hindered if he has already had conventional treatment.

Macrobiotic diets vary according to the type of cancer being "treated" and who recommends it, but for the most part they are vegetarian diets. The American Dietetic Association recognizes that a vegetarian diet may be adequate for many people, and they provide excellent guidelines for planning such diets. But the macrobiotic diets are often deficient in nutrients such as vitamins C and D, caloric energy, and iron. The most restrictive of the macrobiotic diets can lead to scurvy, anemia, abnormally low blood protein, calcium deficiency, loss of kidney function due to low fluid intake, and emaciation due to starvation. Needless to say, the cancer patient needs all the nutrition and strength he can get.

After careful study, the American Cancer Society published an article that stated no evidence had been found that treatment with macrobiotic diets could result in *any* benefit to cancer patients, and they strongly warned against them. The ACS pointed out that the more restrictive macrobiotic diets pose a serious hazard to one's health.

Despite some convincing personal narratives by patients who claim to have been helped, it is most likely they were responding to earlier treatment or are in natural remission.

In addition to the physical damage that can occur from this type of diet, untold numbers suffer deep psychological pain at being told they brought the cancer upon themselves because of their premacrobiotic life-styles. Such a notion is groundless and damaging.

Immuno-Augmentative Therapy

Many people have gone to a clinic in the Bahamas where a variety of cancers was treated with an agent, referred to as IAT, derived from various parts of human blood. Patients were treated briefly and then sent home with large supplies of serum for further injections. The director of the clinic reported great success but refused to support these findings sufficiently for publication in any reputable, professional journal. He also has not published details of the method of preparing the material used.

In 1985 the National Centers for Disease Control, in the United States, announced that patients who received the above drug were exposing themselves to a virus associated with hepatitis and AIDS, and were at risk for both. Even before this, the American Cancer Society had stated that the treatment showed no evidence of any benefit in treatment of human cancers.

The clinic was closed in 1985 by the Bahamian Health Ministry, but a similar setup may reappear elsewhere.

Meditation

Intensive meditation can make many people feel better. But no studies have ever demonstrated that transcendental meditation (TM), mind healing, or any system that enables you to have an experience of deep mental relaxation will cure cancer. Meditation *can* improve the quality of life, but it would be dangerous to accept it as a substitute for treatment, or to feel that "I didn't meditate correctly or enough" if your condition doesn't improve.

Biofeedback

Biofeedback is an excellent medical tool that provides people with visual or auditory information about some of the involuntary functions of the body, such as blood pressure, muscle tension, pulse and respiration rates, and brain-wave activity. Biofeedback usually is a medically safe and painless learning process that, using trial and error, allows people to consciously control certain functions that were once regarded as purely involuntary. Biofeedback is very successful in treating or controlling conditions such as hypertension, migraine headaches, insomnia, certain circulatory disorders, and digestive disorders. It can be helpful for many people with pain. By itself, biofeedback *cannot* cure cancer (or other diseases), despite some quack claims to that effect, but it can be effective in learning to relax.

Mental Imagery

"Close your eyes, and imagine your white cells in a hand-to-hand combat with the cancer cells. The chemotherapy or radiation you are receiving is making the white cells grow stronger by the minute, and as you cheer them on, they slowly but surely destroy every one of the cancer cells. After completing the job, the white cells do not triumphantly quit but remain powerful and vigilant. They perform as sentries, preventing any cancer cells from sneaking past your ally, the immune system. *You* are the commander-in-chief, alert and strong, always aware of danger lurking, but refusing to allow the fierce opposition from cowering you into submission."

Imagery like this, or variations thereof, can be enormously helpful to a cancer patient's attitude toward being cured. One person receiving chemotherapy or radiation may visualize the drugs or X rays as guided missiles that can destroy even invisible cancer cells. Another may picture his body like a giant video game screen; the little Pac-Men are gobbling up the cancer cells.

One patient said he liked to imagine he was sitting on the bank of a brook. He is slowly, methodically tossing stones into the water. Each stone hits the spot to which a water snake is trying to return. Collectively, the stones keep the snake from approaching. This man imagines the water snake as the primary cancer, the snake's attempt to return as a recurrence, and the stones as the treatment.

Many people, without ever having read or even heard about the technique of "guided imagery," spontaneously conjure up images like these. It gives them a sense of control over their treatment and disease.

So far, so good. Anything that makes it easier to cope with treatment helps you achieve a positive outlook and a sense of control is useful, *if* you continue with your medical treatment. Many experts believe that an active, positive attitude about your own care *may* increase the effectiveness of treatment.

Unfortunately, many (but certainly not *all*) proponents of these guided-imagery techniques take the attitude that you, the patient, are solely responsible for your own return to health. They recommend you go through a complex program involving an appraisal of the stresses in your life that preceded cancer, of how *you* participated in those stresses, and how you are now "benefiting" from becoming ill. They claim that only by confronting these stresses and the maladaptive way in which you seem to handle them can you change your behavior *and* get well.

It is always a good idea to change maladaptive behavior, because this can have a positive effect on such stress-related ailments as tension headaches and muscle pains. But in the opinion of most oncologists, psychiatrists, nurses, and social workers, anyone who tells you that it is possible to "think away your cancer" (with *or* without conventional treatment) is harshly deceiving you.

One patient described her experience:

It was bad enough to get cancer, but then to hear it was my fault was even worse. I was devastated when a "counselor" at the program said that I chose (yes, you heard me right, he said *chose*) to develop cancer because I had negative emotions. He said these emotions were experienced biologically at the level of the cell and *that* had caused the cancer.

So even though I couldn't turn back the clock, I did everything they told me to do in the program that would help me get well again. I tried to build up my immunity defenses with images of the drugs working to melt away the cancer. I went through the entire program, at great financial cost, as though my life depended upon it. I believed that my life depended upon the program as much, if not more, than on the drugs.

And then I had a recurrence. Now I'm getting radiation and my oncologist says he believes I will do well. The recurrence filled me with an overwhelming sense of failure. Not only did I have to deal with the recurrence of the cancer as a life-threatening experience, but I was so burdened with self-reproach and guilt that I could barely function. I blamed myself for not being able to do anything right. At that point I wondered if life was worth living.

Fortunately, this woman saw an excellent psychiatrist who specializes in treating cancer patients. Later she joined a cancer support group led by an experienced social worker. She was luckier than others who are made to suffer emotionally without the support of psychiatrists, social workers, and other caring people. Still others forgo conventional treatment that could have helped them. They rely *only* on programs or so-called therapists who teach them how to rid their body of cancer by way of various mental imageries.

Although many studies have indicated that there is a direct relationship between stress and the development of cancer, others dispute this theory. Some experts say that the stress may be the result of cancer, not the cause of it. And although some studies have shown that a feisty, angry attitude toward disease can lead to increased survival, other studies do not.

Imagery, visualization, and other similar therapies can be extremely helpful when coordinated with your overall treatment, especially in coping with the disease and its treatment.

But stay away from anything that:

- claims to cure your cancer without any other treatment.
- claims to cure your cancer with the *addition* of their "secret drug."
- tells you that you brought on, or chose to develop, cancer.
- says that you are choosing not to get better.

- implies that your attitude is keeping you from getting better.
- promises that this technique has cured a number of people whom conventional doctors had "given up" on.

Why Do Some of These Unproven Methods Sometimes "Work"?

Unproven methods are not merely—unproven, they have clearly *proved to be ineffective.* Yet some patients do seem to improve, even if only temporarily. Why?

Often the patients are responding to conventional treatment received prior to these methods. Other times they never received an accurate diagnosis to begin with. Sometimes their disease is the kind that has plateaus (periods of time in which the cancer is stable, neither improving nor getting worse). Occasionally a spontaneous remission occurs. And rarely—but it does happen—spontaneous cure occurs.

But some patients truly do respond to even the most ineffective treatment. Is there an explanation?

The Placebo Effect

You have probably heard about placebos. A placebo is an inactive substance prescribed as if it were an effective medication. Placebos are used to study the effect of some medications, and are sometimes prescribed by doctors for patients whom they feel have "imaginary" (that is, psychologically caused) symptoms. Formerly, researchers claimed that the reason many placebos appear to succeed is simply that some illnesses get better with or without a drug.

But anthropologists have long noted that some folk medicine actually works because people believe it will work. When physicians learned about endorphins and other chemicals that the body forms, which act on the central and peripheral nervous systems to reduce pain, they began to understand the success of placebos. When stimulated to do so, the brain produces endorphins, which are similar to morphine and can, like morphine, reduce pain. The body also produces epinephrine, which reduces inflammations and congestion, and interferon, which has been shown (see Chapter 7) to have an effect in certain circumstances against cancer cells.

Today we know that the body and brain work together in remarkable ways. Belief has a powerful effect on all people, including the most highly educated. Whether the belief is in a shaman's magic, the surgeon's scalpel, the faith healer's words and touch, standard chemotherapy drugs, *or* the quack's medications, the placebo effect may be in operation.

But belief alone is insufficient to cure cancer. You need every weapon available, and conventional medicine offers the best and most powerful ones.

Quackery, Pure and Simple

There will always be unscrupulous and misguided people who exploit cancer patients. Some are only looking for an easy dollar. Others may really believe in what they are doing. They often have a fine-looking office with leather chairs, a mahogany desk, diplomas and certificates hanging on the wall. They wear white coats and have polished speech, using words like clinic, therapy, diagnosis, prognosis. They talk of studies and protocols. And they usually take time to listen to you, something your own physician doesn't always do.

But no matter what their approach, the end result is the same: Those for whom cure was available by way of conventional treatment lose that opportunity. Others get short-changed on length and quality of survival. Patients may become geographically or emotionally distanced from family and friends, and they spend a great deal of money that cannot be reimbursed by insurance. It is, undoubtedly, the ultimate and cruelest con game. The American Cancer Society maintains an updated list of materials on unproven methods of cancer management, available from their national office. It includes lists of drugs and other substances, organizations, health centers, books, magazines and newsletters.

If you have any questions about any treatment, call the ACS or the National Cancer Institute.

Section Three

TYPES OF CANCER

Chapter 9
Specific Cancers: Symptoms, Diagnosis, and Treatment

Cancer is described both by type of cells and by their location; treatment varies accordingly. In this chapter I will try to give you an overview of some broad categories of cancers: their symptoms, diagnosis, and treatment. Please refer to earlier chapters for full explanations of diagnostic techniques and treatments. In Section Four, I will describe some of the ways you can cope with both the disease itself and the various treatments.

Within each of the broad categories listed below are some specific cancers; discussion follows of the most common types. In Appendix VII, you will find some books that discuss in full some of the cancers listed here. In addition, your local librarian—or perhaps your doctor or nurse—may be able to refer you to some of the latest journal articles on treatment for your particular kind of cancer. The National Cancer Institute is probably your very best "hot line"; they will refer you to the latest information on diagnosis and treatment. The American Cancer Society also publishes material on specific cancers. Call the nearest division or unit; they are listed in your phone book.

CANCERS OF THE HEAD AND NECK

Cancers of the head and neck include those of the lip, oral cavity (including tongue, mouth, cheek), tonsils, salivary glands, sinuses, nasal cavities, and larynx. People who use tobacco (including pipes, cigars, chewing tobacco, as well as cigarettes) or consume a great deal of alcohol are at high risk for these cancers. The use of both substances together produces an even greater risk.

Thyroid cancer, another head-and-neck cancer, is closely associated with radiation exposure, whose effects may take decades to surface. At one time (before such treatment was found to be harmful), many children and adolescents were given X-ray treatment for acne, tonsil infections, earaches, and even excess facial hair. As adults, these people are at risk for developing cancer of the thyroid. Fortunately, it is highly curable when treated early.

Cancer of the larynx (laryngeal cancer). The larynx, or voice box, is the upper portion of the windpipe, containing the vocal cords. When you breathe, air enters the nose or mouth and passes through the larynx into your lungs. A small structure overhangs the larynx like a lid, closing when you swallow, to prevent food from entering the larynx. Air passing through the larynx causes the vocal cords to vibrate, permitting sound to be produced.

An early symptom of cancer of the larynx is prolonged hoarseness, which is usually caused by a tumor originating on the vocal cords. A change in voice pitch, a lump in the throat, coughing, difficulty or pain in breathing or swallowing, or even an earache may be an early symptom of a tumor in areas above or below the vocal cords. In these instances, hoarseness may develop later, or not at all.

Most tumors of the larynx can be detected with a medical examination using a small mirror with a long handle and an examination of the lymph nodes. X rays and a laryngoscopy (which allows the doctor to look at the tumor and remove a portion of tissue for biopsy) are used for diagnosis of the tumor's type, size, and extent of growth.

Radiation therapy is used to treat and cure most small or early tumors. Larger tumors are surgically removed in a procedure called a *laryngectomy*. If the doctor performs a partial laryngectomy, the patient will be left with a normal or slightly hoarse voice. In a total laryngectomy, the entire larynx is removed, and the pharynx is closed so that food can be swallowed normally. The upper trachea is stitched to an opening in the skin so that air can pass through this "tracheostomy" and enter the lungs. Patients then breathe through this opening, or stomas, rather than through the nose and mouth.

In the event of a total laryngectomy, the patient can learn to speak again through a technique known as esophageal speech. (See Chapter 10 for further information.)

When the cancer has spread beyond the larynx, other, more extensive surgery may be required, including a "neck dissection," which involves the surgical removal of the lymph nodes and surrounding structures within the neck.

In addition to surgery and radiation, chemotherapy is used to treat cancer of the larynx.

Leukoplakia: A precancerous condition. White patches or red, inflamed areas in the mouth are often indicative of this condition, which may *precede* cancer of the tongue, lip, and floor of the mouth. A dentist may first notice it and will send a patient to an otolaryngologist (ear, nose, and throat surgeon) for a full evaluation.

Cancer of the mouth and oral cavity (oral cancer). This cancer may be located on the floor of the mouth, the pharynx (including the soft palate), the lips, or the tongue. Cancer can also develop in the salivary glands, the gums, the hard palate (roof of the mouth), and the buccal mucosa (the soft tissues inside the cheeks).

A sore; a raised growth, swelling, or lump; changes in tissue color; continuous bleeding, tingling, burning, or numbness; difficulty in swallowing or talking; and any other discomfort that persists in the mouth for more than ten days are all symptoms of oral cancer. An evaluation by a dentist or physician may include a biopsy of any suspicious areas.

Surgery may include the removal of nearby lymph glands in addition to the tumor. Radiation may be offered instead of, or as well as, surgery. Both external and internal radiation (interstitial irradiation) are used to treat many mouth cancers. Chemotherapy is also indicated in many instances.

Surgery in and around the mouth may be disfiguring, but through the latest techniques in reconstructive surgery, doctors can rebuild facial features and minimize cosmetic defects. (This procedure will be discussed further in Chapter 10.)

Cancer of the thyroid. The thyroid gland, located in front of the neck under the Adam's apple, is part of the endocrine system and is essential to normal body growth in infancy and childhood.

The first symptoms of thyroid cancer may be hardly perceptible; you may notice some mild swelling low in the neck only because your collars seem tight, or your physician may see something during a routine physical examination. Later symptoms may include difficulty in breathing or swallowing, hoarseness, or a hard lump.

A thyroid scan and ultrasound are the chief tools of diagnosis. Your doctor may also perform chest X rays, X rays of the neck, and a laryngoscopy, to see if the cancer has spread.

Treatment for very early abnormalities of the thyroid may be limited to oral doses of hormones. Cancer of the thyroid gland is treated by surgical removal of part or all of the gland, and sometimes of nearby lymph glands as well. If all of the thyroid gland is removed, you will have to take a thyroid replacement, in pill form, for the remainder of your life. When only a portion of the thyroid is removed, such replacement may not be necessary.

Other, less common head-and-neck cancers are treated with surgery, radiation, or a combination of both, and sometimes with chemotherapy. Treatment of any of these cancers should be performed by a physician who specializes in head-and-neck surgery. Otolaryngologists, general surgeons, and plastic surgeons do head and neck surgery. Be sure your surgeon is board-certified in one of those specialties and is a member of the American Society for Head and Neck Surgery or the Society of Head and Neck Surgeons. Their membership in the societies will be listed in the *Directory of Specialists*, which is described on page 000.

CANCER OF THE LUNG

The lungs are two spongy, pinkish-gray organs that are the center of the respiratory system, enabling you to breathe. The left lung has two sections, known as lobes. The right lung is slightly larger and has three lobes. When you breathe, the air you inhale through your mouth or nose goes through the trachea, which divides into the two bronchus tubes (the bronchi), then into the bronchioles, tiny branches of air tubes in the lung. Through these tubes, the air reaches the alveoli, tiny air sacs or clusters, which pass the oxygen on to the bloodstream.

Most lung cancers begin in the bronchi or bronchioles, and for this reason are also called bronchogenic cancers. It is believed that lung cancers may develop slowly over a period of twenty or more years. Industrial exposure to carcinogens such as asbestos, arsenic, chromium, radiation, uranium, certain chemicals and petroleum products increase one's risk of developing lung cancer, but smoking is the most common cause. Smoking also increases the risk of developing cancer in those who have been exposed to other carcinogens. Yet not every heavy smoker gets lung cancer. And many people develop lung cancer who do not smoke and are unable to recall specific exposure to any carcinogens.

The most common symptoms of lung cancer are:

- Coughing, which develops when a growing cancer blocks an airway. The cough may have recently developed or be a worsening of a chronic condition.

- Blood: coughing up blood, or sputum (expectorated matter, including saliva and discharged substances from respiratory passages) that is streaked with rust-colored or bright red blood.
- Chest pain: a persistent ache that may or may not be related to a cough.
- Unexplained fever or infection.
- Wheezing, shortness of breath, or hoarseness.
- Pneumonia or bronchitis; particularly recurring bouts of it.
- Fatigue, loss of appetite, and weight loss.

The conventional, routine chest X ray seldom detects early lung cancer. Thus, when lung cancer is diagnosed, it may be fairly advanced. The best prevention is not to smoke, but for those who do, some experts recommend they have a sputum test yearly. In this test, a laboratory examination is made of your sputum to see if cancer cells are present. Test results are not, however, always accurate.

When a physician suspects lung cancer, he will begin the diagnostic process with a chest X ray, sputum test, and blood tests, and then may also arrange for you to have tomograms or CAT scans. He might also arrange for:

- A *bronchoscopy,* in which the fiber-optic instrument is inserted through the nose or mouth and threaded into the branches of the lung airways for viewing and for removal of tissue for biopsy (an outpatient procedure).
- A *needle biopsy,* in which tissue is removed through a needle inserted into the chest. A pleural biopsy is done with a large needle, through which a piece of pleural tissue as well as fluid is removed (an outpatient procedure).
- A *mediastinoscopy,* in which the instrument is inserted through a small incision in the neck near the breastbone and passed through into the mediastinum, the area between the lungs and behind the breastbone. This test permits examination and biopsy of the lymph nodes near the lung (an inpatient procedure).
- A *mediastinotomy,* which is similar to the above procedure except that the incision is made either to the right or left side of the breastbone (an inpatient procedure).
- A *thorascopy,* which is performed in the operating room under general anesthesia. This test is done when others have been inconclusive. An incision is made between the ribs, and the lung is deflated so that it and the surrounding structures can be examined. A biopsy is obtained and the lung is then reinflated (an inpatient procedure).

In some instances, a *thoracotomy* may be done for a complete and definitive diagnosis. This is a major surgical procedure, consisting of opening the chest and conducting a complete and careful examination of the lungs and chest cavity. If the surgeon finds cancerous growth that is confined to one lung, part or all of it may be removed.

Prior to treatment, lung cancer is fully staged to determine its extent. This may be done after the bronchoscopy, but before a thoracotomy is planned. The stage of the disease and the cell type are important factors in determining the correct treatment.

There are a number of types of cancer that begin in the lung. These four major types account for almost all lung cancers:

- *Epidermoid, or squamous-cell, carcinoma.* Arises from cells that line the airways. Tends to remain localized in the chest for longer periods than other cell types.
- *Large-cell carcinoma.* Has large, rounded cells. Tends to grow in secondary or smaller bronchi.
- *Small-cell carcinoma* (also called *oat-cell carcinoma* because of the cell shape). Tends to spread early. This cancer is *never* treated surgically, but always with chemotherapy and sometimes radiation.
- *Adenocarcinoma.* Originates and frequently grows under the inner lining of the air passages of the lung.

Surgical removal of one lung or a portion of it is the treatment for a certain amount of early lung cancers. Nearby lymph nodes may be removed as well. The removal of one lobe is called a *lobectomy*; removal of an entire lung is called a *pneumonectomy*. If the cancer has spread beyond the lung, surgery is not performed. Lung cancers are also treated with radiation and/or chemotherapy. Radiation is also used for palliation, to relieve cough, pain, shortness of breath, or difficulty in swallowing.

Pulmonary specialists do many of the diagnostic tests for lung cancer; thoracic surgeons perform surgical procedures. Your primary physician may be a medical oncologist or pulmonary specialist.

BREAST CANCER

It was not until the 1970s—when President Ford's wife, Betty Ford, talked openly of her mastectomy—that breast cancer really came out into the open. Suddenly, it was widely written about and discussed.

Although breast cancer does occur in men, it is rare, amounting to less than 1,000 cases a year in this country. In American women, however, it represents more than one quarter of all cancers, approximately 119,000 a year.

Who is at risk? Those women at high risk for cancer have a close-family history of breast cancer—usually involving a mother, sister, aunt, grandmother, or even daughter—and their risk is increased if their relatives developed it prior to menopause. The risk is also higher-than-average for women who began menstruating early, had a late menopause, had their first child after thirty, or have had no children at all. A high-fat diet and weight gain also contribute to high risk. And there has been speculation that women who took diethylstilbestrol (DES)—a drug once prescribed during pregnancy for some women who habitually miscarried—may be at high risk for breast cancer.

An estimated 10 to 15 percent of those women who have had cancer in one breast will develop it in the other.

Breast cancer is the cancer that women fear most. And no wonder. The average woman has one chance in eleven of developing breast cancer during her lifetime. Although symptoms may throw a woman into panic, it is important to remember that in nine out of every ten cases in which some abnormality is found in a breast, it turns out to be harmless. Still, *no* symptom of breast cancer should be ignored. Early detection and early treatment can save your life—and sometimes your breast as well.

Symptoms

All women should learn and then practice monthly breast self-examination (BSE). Many hospitals and community health centers sponsor "teach-ins" where you can learn, and some family physicians and gynecologists instruct their patients or arrange for a nurse to do it. During BSE you will look for any irregularities or lumps; if you find any, report them immediately to your physician for further evaluation.

Often a breast lump is one of these benign conditions:

- *Cystic disease:* fluid-filled sacs that enlarge and become tender. Usually found near the armpit and are movable (slide around under the skin). Most common in women thirty-five to fifty years old.
- *Lipomas:* slow-growing, soft, movable lumps usually found in postmenopausal women.
- *Traumatic fat necrosis:* painless, round, firm lumps caused by fat in breast that may have arisen from a minor bruise. Most often appears in older women and in women with very large breasts.

- *Fibroadenomas:* painless, firm, rubbery, movable, and lumps, often oval in shape. Most often found in women fifteen to thirty years old.

A woman cannot evaluate these or other changes by herself or determine if they are truly symptoms of breast cancer. Although natural changes in a woman's breast are caused by such factors as age, menstrual cycle, pregnancy, breast-feeding, birth-control or other hormone pills, menopause, a bruise or blow to the breast, they should never be ignored. *Over 70 percent of all breast cancers are found by women themselves.*

Any of the following symptoms may also be significant and could indicate cancer of the breast:

- Lump or thickening in the breast.
- Discharge from the nipple.
- Scaliness of the skin, especially around the nipple.
- Change in color or texture of the skin.
- Sudden or gradual change of any kind, unrelated to menstrual cycle.
- An enlargement of a gland (node) in the armpit (rare but nevertheless possible).
- "Dimpling" or "puckering" of skin on or in the region of the breast.

A woman would be wise to follow the American Cancer Society guidelines on mammography. At age forty, she should have a "baseline" mammogram. If she has a family history of breast cancer or any other high-risk factor, she should have this done at thirty-five. This is considered a screening device and can detect any abnormalities that may be present. If the mammogram is normal, it can be kept on file to compare with later, routine X rays. Mammography is fully described on pages 000–000.

Diagnosis

Most women who suspect some breast abnormality initially see their gynecologist or family physician. Some may decide to consult with a breast surgeon. The physician will take a full history and palpate the breasts, using his hands to feel the tissues. He may order a sonogram, thermogram, or use a strong light to perform transillumination. These methods are not reliable enough to be used alone, so he will very likely recommend mammography or the diagnostic procedures of aspiration and biopsy.

Your doctor may send you for a mammogram even if you had one recently. This is more a detection than a diagnostic test and is done to identify any abnormalities that he may suspect and to determine changes that have occurred since you had a baseline mammogram.

Aspiration can be done in the surgeon's office. By inserting a fine hypodermic needle into the lump, he can determine whether a lump is fluid-filled or is a solid mass. If the lump is a fluid-filled cyst, it will collapse as he withdraws the fluid. The fluid will be analyzed in a laboratory; if it is bloody or contains suspicious cells, further diagnostic procedures will be performed.

If the lump is a solid mass, the physician can, with a different kind of needle, remove a bit of tissue for laboratory analysis. This type of biopsy, known as an *incisional biopsy* (see page 25), is not by any means definitive. The laboratory report is sometimes a "false negative," which means that the particular specimen removed and examined had no malignancy cells in it simply because the needle "missed" them.

If your physician suspects cancer, based on any of the office or outpatient procedures described, he may want you to have a more thorough biopsy, rather than rely on an *incisional* biopsy alone. Depending on the size of the mass, your general condition, and other factors, this may be an outpatient procedure done with a local anesthetic or performed in a hospital under general anesthesia.

Since most women call a lump to the attention of their doctor while it is still small, removal of the entire mass for diagnosis (called an *excisional biopsy*) is seldom a disfiguring procedure. Thus, most experts now believe that the entire mass should be cut out surgically so that it can be thoroughly and completely examined.

Separating diagnosis and treatment. Until the 1970s, diagnosis and treatment were usually merged into one procedure. If a physician suspected that a woman had breast cancer, she was scheduled for a "one-step procedure." She was admitted to the hospital, taken to the operating room, anesthetized, and a biopsy was performed. If the frozen section (see page 25) indicated cancer, the surgeon performed a mastectomy—removal of the breast and a great deal of the surrounding area.

Rose Kushner, a medical writer, told of her own breast-cancer experiences in her book *Why Me?* (see Appendix VII). In 1974, she had to search hard for a doctor who would agree to schedule *only* a biopsy of her breast lump. She wished, on the basis of the results of a permanent section (more reliable than a frozen section) to discuss the treatment plan with her physicians. She finally found such a doctor, and after her two-step procedure she fought in the press, at the National Cancer Institute, and with individual oncologists so that *all* women could have the opportunity she had demanded and received. Today the two-step, or "two-stage," operation is widely recommended by oncologists and surgeons. It is now known that waiting a short period of time between biopsy and mastectomy does not affect treatment outcome.

However, some women prefer the one-step procedure, and tell their physicians that if cancer is found during a hospital biopsy they wish to have any necessary surgery performed then and there. But every woman is entitled to a choice, and if her doctor will not agree to a two-step procedure, she should and will be able to find someone else who will. As I'll explain a bit later, some studies indicate that in many instances it is possible to have effective treatment of cancer with removal of the malignant lump only, followed by radiation. As a matter of fact, in some states it is now a law that physicians explain this to patients when their treatment is discussed.

If on the basis of a biopsy—or any other part of the diagnostic procedure—cancer is found in the breast, further staging follows to determine its extent. Staging should be completed after biopsy but *before* any other surgical procedure.

Because breast cancer can spread to the bones, liver, lungs, and brain, your doctor will order various scans and X rays to determine if there is any spread beyond the glands in the armpit. Most important, he will arrange for *estrogen-* and *progesterone-receptor assays* to be done of the malignant mass. These tests determine if the cancer will respond to hormonal treatments, and which ones will work best. The estrogen-receptor assay (ERA) is done routinely today, but the progesterone assay (PRA) is new and may not be available everywhere. In the opinion of most experts, it *should* be done for all breast-cancer patients. Your doctor should arrange for these tests prior to biopsy, because the malignant tissue must be frozen within fifteen minutes of its removal from the breast, especially if it is to be sent to a laboratory outside the hospital.

Even if hormonal treatment is not indicated shortly after surgery, it may be at some later date, and the information obtained from the assays will be of major importance.

Treating Breast Cancer

Proper treatment for breast cancer varies and, according to some experts, is still a controversial issue. However, there seems to be general agreement that if the cancer has spread throughout the body, a mastectomy is unnecessary.

Generally, treatment for breast cancer consists of one of the procedures listed below—dependent upon many factors. In some instances, the "jury is still out" on which is the optimum treatment, so your physician may present you with alternatives and let you decide. You would be wise to seek a second opinion, regardless of the recommendation or options presented.

At one time breast cancer was treated almost exclusively by mastectomy. The *Halsted radical mastectomy*—in which the breast, all underlying muscles, and lymph nodes were removed in a debilitating procedure—was once standard treatment, but it is no longer recommended by most major cancer centers. The NCI stated in 1979 that a ten-year study showed that there was no difference in survival rates between those who had had the Halsted radical and those who had had the modified radical mastectomy.

The modified radical mastectomy traditionally consisted of the removal of the breast alone. Nowadays it is sometimes also called *total mastectomy with axillary dissection*. During this procedure, the breast, underarm lymph nodes, and the lining over the chest muscles are removed. Sometimes two small chest muscles are also removed. It is the most frequent treatment for early-stage breast cancer.

Total, or simple, mastectomy is a procedure during which only the breast is removed. Sometimes a few of the underarm lymph nodes closest to the breast are removed, to see if the cancer has spread beyond the breast.

Partial mastectomy, or segmental resection (sometimes called a lumpectomy, though not exactly the same thing), is the removal of the tumor plus a wedge of normal tissue surrounding it. Some of the skin and the lining of the chest muscle below the tumor is also removed. Some or all of the underarm lymph nodes may be removed to determine if the cancer has spread.

Lumpectomy is the removal of the breast lump plus a margin of normal tissue around it. This procedure is usually followed by radiation therapy.

There is a distinct difference between a modified or total mastectomy and a lumpectomy, but some of the other procedures seem to overlap, and the same procedures may be differently labeled by some surgeons. You should ask the surgeon to describe the procedure rather than simply give it a title. It also should be noted that a lumpectomy in a small breast may, cosmetically, appear not much different from a mastectomy.

Removal of some tissue from the underarm lymph nodes is essential to determine if the cancer has spread, regardless of the surgical procedure performed.

Depending on the findings, surgery for breast cancer may be followed by chemotherapy (combined chemotherapy and/or hormonal manipulation) and/or radiation. Radiation may be internal or external, as explained in Chapter 5.

A National Cancer Institute–sponsored study reported in early 1985 that some early cancers can be treated as successfully with *segmental resection* and radiation to the breast as with mastectomy. It has been estimated that due to early detection almost half of the women who develop breast cancer might be candidates for this procedure. But critics of the report say that the study, begun in 1976, is not conclusive, because some breast cancers recur still later. Others also remind patients that since lumpectomy followed by radiotherapy to the intact breast has only recently become a standard procedure, they should make sure that their surgeon is very familiar and experienced at doing it. They caution that only a radiotherapist who is very experienced in radiating the intact breast will be able to avoid effects that may be as (or even more) cosmetically disfiguring as mastectomy.

Discussion with physicians from each specialty. It would be wise to consult with a medical oncologist and a radiotherapist in addition to a surgeon, and to obtain a second surgical opinion *prior* to surgery. Remember: *No woman has to agree to a one-stage operation, a procedure in which she is put to sleep and doesn't know whether she's going to wake up with or without her breast.* And she may have other options; *surgery is not the only treatment for all breast cancers.*

Some communities and hospitals, recognizing the need for women to seek out and confer with a number of physicians in order to weigh their advice, have formed a collaborative breast service where patients seeking second opinions can come to explore and learn more about the treatment options available to them. Patients can see an oncologist, breast surgeon, and radiotherapist, often at the same time. These experts will confer with each other, as well as with the patient, outline her options and/or make recommendations. In time, this kind of collaborative service may become more widely available.

Mastectomy has a profound emotional effect on women—in addition to the general feelings about having cancer. Many women choose to have plastic surgery, in which the breast is reconstructed after surgery. I will discuss these aspects of breast cancer in Chapter 10. It would be wise to discuss the possibility of reconstruction with your surgeon *prior* to mastectomy, because he may wish to make certain advance preparations.

Initial diagnosis of breast cancer is often made by a woman's family physician or gynecologist. A general surgeon can perform breast surgery, but he should be well trained and experienced in breast surgery and surgical oncology. He may very well be a member of one of the clinical oncological societies. A medical oncologist should also follow up on the patient after surgery.

CANCERS OF THE UPPER DIGESTIVE TRACT

The upper digestive tract includes those organs, structures, and glands through which food passes from the mouth and breaks down in preparation for absorption into the bloodstream before carrying waste to the intestines for excretion.

Cancers of the upper digestive tract include those of the esophagus, stomach, liver, and pancreas as well as the rarer ones of the gallbladder and small intestine. (Those of the large intestine and rectum will be considered under a separate section, immediately following this one.)

These organs are located deep in the body and are not readily accessible to examination during routine medical checkups. Cancers in this area may be a long time in developing, but they remain "silent," showing no symptoms until they have grown to a considerable size.

Cancer of the esophagus. The esophagus is the narrow, muscular ten-inch tube that carries food and liquids from the throat to the stomach. Cancer of the esophagus is more common in men than in women and most often develops in those who are heavy users of tobacco (whether smoked or chewed).

Difficulty in swallowing is the most common early symptom of esophageal cancer. A sticking sensation somewhere behind the breastbone may be felt, whether or not food is actually stuck. There may be a burning sensation or persistent pain. Because of the difficulty in swallowing, eating becomes difficult and the patient may lose weight.

Diagnosis is usually made by means of an X ray of the esophagus, after swallowing barium; and an esophagoscopy, in which the doctor can examine the esophagus and take a tissue sample for biopsy. Further scans and tests may be done to see if the cancer has spread.

The principle methods of treatment are external radiation and/or surgery. The decision is made, in part, according to the location of the tumor. Surgery is done under general anesthesia, usually by a gastrointestinal surgeon or a thoracic surgeon, but many general surgeons also do the procedure. The surgeon usually begins by making an incision between the ribs on the afflicted side of the chest. The malignant area is removed and the healthy area reconnected to the stomach, sometimes with a plastic tube. Occasionally a tube is inserted directly into the stomach through the abdominal wall, permitting pureed food and food supplements to be fed to the patient.

Treatment may also include chemotherapy. Your case will be followed by a gastroenterologist and/or medical oncologist.

Cancer of the stomach. The stomach is the major organ of digestion and is located in the upper right area of the abdomen. Food and liquids are funneled from the mouth and esophagus into the stomach, where they are partially processed before moving on to the intestines.

The incidence of stomach (or gastric) cancer is higher in men than in women, seldom developing before age forty and usually not until sixty or so. Those at highest risk are people with a relative who has had the disease, those with atrophic gastritis (chronic inflammation of the stomach lining), failure to produce gastric juices, and pernicious anemia. People whose diet is high in smoked, pickled, and salted food may also be at risk.

The first symptom is often vague digestive discomfort. Unfortunately, this is often ignored by physician and patient alike. Further symptoms—such as lack of appetite, weight loss, or severe anemia—usually lead to further investigation. Diagnosis involves analysis of the stool for hidden blood, an upper GI series, and cytological examination of cells shed from the stomach. Through fiber-optic gastroscopy, the physician can view the stomach and take a tissue sample for analysis.

Cancer of the stomach is usually treated by surgical removal of part or all of the stomach. Despite the diagnostic tests, it is sometimes difficult, prior to surgery, to differentiate between a malignant stomach tumor and a benign stomach ulcer. If it is cancer and has spread to adjacent organs such as the spleen, pancreas, or colon, these may also be removed. This is major surgery, of course, and should be performed by an abdominal or general surgeon who is experienced in the procedure.

It is possible to live a normal life without a stomach, but you will have to eat smaller, more frequent meals, and maintain a high-protein, low-sugar diet.

After surgery, you should also be followed up on by a gastroenterologist and/or a medical oncologist. Radiation and chemotherapy may also be offered.

Cancer of the pancreas. The pancreas is a large gland that stretches across the abdominal wall behind the stomach. It secretes two essential substances. One is the hormone insulin, which regulates the amount of sugar in the blood. The other is pancreatic juice, which contains enzymes that aid in the digestion of food.

At highest risk for pancreatic cancer are diabetics and those who smoke or drink heavily. The first symptom of cancer of the pancreas may be a vague pain in the upper abdomen, sometimes spreading to the back. It may be intermittent, gradually becoming persistent. Other symptoms are nausea, loss of appetite, weight loss, and general weakness, often varying according to the precise location of the tumor. Depression is often associated with cancer of the pancreas.

Diagnosis begins with laboratory tests of blood, urine, and stool, and an upper GI series. The doctor may also arrange for angiograms, radioactive scanning, ultrasound, and/or CAT scans. Definitive diagnosis will probably be made by a biopsy. Some new tests allow tissue samples to be taken with a fiber-optic instrument, but often surgery through the abdomen is the only way to reach the pancreas.

Treatment may include surgical removal of the tumor alone, or of the entire pancreas. Any other areas blocked may also be removed. If the pancreas is removed, prescribed medications will assume the pancreatic functions. Chemotherapy and radiation may be offered as treatment.

Cancer of the liver. The liver is the largest gland of the body and one of its most complex because it has so many functions. It secretes bile, which helps in absorption of fat and prevents jaundice, and is essential to various metabolic processes. The presence of the liver is essential for life, but it can continue to function even if most of it is removed.

Most cancers of the liver are secondary tumors that have spread from another site. Primary cancer of the liver is very rare in the United States. Those at highest risk are people who have been exposed to vinyl chloride at work (such as plastic workers), and athletes who have taken synthetic testosterone, a male hormone that promotes muscle development. Also at risk are those who have suffered from cirrhosis of the liver, a chronic degenerative disease which follows severe nutritional deprivation, hepatitis, or some other infection; or develops as a result of chronic alcohol abuse.

Early signs and symptoms of liver cancer are often silent; when noticeable, they include: vague pain in the right upper portion of the abdomen, weakness, tiredness, weight loss, discomfort on deep breathing and coughing, pain in the shoulder toward the back. If the tumor is obstructing the bile duct, jaundice (yellowing of skin) may develop.

A diagnostic workup will include a nuclear liver scan, CAT scan, endoscopy, and other visual examinations; a needle biopsy; and various blood studies. These tests also help to determine if the tumor is a primary or secondary one, and to stage the disease.

Surgery can be performed to remove tumors and even a portion of the liver if the cancer is localized in one lobe. Unfortunately, however, the entire liver cannot be removed (unless a transplant is available), so if the cancer has spread throughout the organ, treatment will depend on chemotherapy and radiation.

Medical care will be provided by a gastroenterologist, general or abdominal surgeon, medical oncologist and/or radiologist.

Cancer of the gallbladder. The gallbladder is attached to the underside of the right lobe of the liver. Its chief function is to serve as a reservoir for bile.

Cancer of the gallbladder is rare, usually developing in older women who have had chronic problems with gallstones. Symptoms are like those for gallstones, including vague to severe abdominal problems. Diagnosis is usually made when surgery is done to treat gallbladder disease. The surgeon removes the gallbladder (this operation is called a *cholecystectomy*), and if the disease has spread to the liver, he will remove part of the liver as well.

Surgery will be performed by a general or abdominal surgeon.

Cancer of the small intestine. The most common symptoms are obstruction, pain, nausea, and vomiting. Diagnosis is made with barium X ray and usually confirmed by surgery, in which a segment of the small intestine is removed.

CANCERS OF THE COLON AND RECTUM

In the summer of 1985 the media spotlight focused on President Ronald Reagan's colon surgery. When newscasters announced that he had colon cancer, much information on his disease was publicized, and the nation's citizens became aware that colorectal cancer afflicts more than 130,000 Americans each year.

The colon and rectum comprise the final segment of the digestive tract. The colon is the major component of the large intestine, or bowel. It is about five to six feet long. The last five or six inches consist of the rectum, which leads to the outside of the body. Solid and semisolid body waste is eliminated through the colon and rectum.

Colorectal cancer (the medical name for cancers of the colon and rectum) affects men and women equally and is most prevalent in those over the age of forty. It is thought that environmental factors—particularly a diet that is high in fat and meat, and low in fiber—play a role in the development of the disease.

Medical experts believe that all cancers of the colorectal area arise from benign polyps, masses of growth protruding from a mucous membrane. This transformation may take years, but removal of a polyp before it becomes malignant can prevent a cancer from developing. People with a history of polyps, ulcerative colitis (ulcers of the colon), or inflammation of the intestines are considered at risk for colorectal cancer. Anyone who has been cured of cancers of the breast or uterus may also be at high risk, as are those whose close family members have had any of the above described problems. If a person has been treated and cured of a cancer of the colon or rectum, they must be watched very closely, because it can recur in other areas of the colon and rectum.

Screening and Early Detection

Screening and early detection are the best prevention. *Everyone* over the age of forty should have a digital rectal examination performed yearly by their physician. At that time, and certainly no later than fifty, one should also begin yearly examinations of the stool for hidden blood. This test, known as a guaiac, or hemoccult, test is a simple one done at home. Several small stool samples are smeared on slides or tabs and then returned to the physician, who sends them to a laboratory for analysis. Similar kits are now available for complete analysis at home. At the age of fifty, everyone should have a proctosigmoidoscope to examine the lower third of the colon. After two successive annual negative examinations, the test need not be repeated for three to five years.

Early colorectal cancer has a high cure rate, thus the American Cancer Society recommends regular screening so that early detection and early treatment are possible. Some gastroenterologists believe that in people at high risk for colorectal cancer, screening should begin at an even younger age than forty and be performed yearly.

Symptoms

When screening and early detection guidelines are closely followed, diagnosis may precede symptoms. Symptoms of colorectal cancer often do not occur until the cancer is fairly well developed; at that time the cure rate is not as good as for early cancers. The most common symptoms of colorectal cancer are:

- Blood in the stool.
- Persistent—lasting two weeks or more—changes in bowel habits, such as alternating diarrhea and constipation.
- Abdominal pain or discomfort.
- Weakness and fatigue (due to anemia from undetectable blood loss).
- Loss of appetite and weight

Diagnosis and Treatment

If blood or any other suspicious signs are evident during screening and detection procedures, a physician will then order diagnostic tests to further rule out the possibility of colorectal cancer.

These tests include a lower GI series and a colonoscopy as well as various blood tests. The colonoscope is a fiber-optic instrument that permits the physician to view the entire colon (rather than just the lower part, as with the proctosigmoidoscope) and to remove samples of suspicious tissues for biopsy. Perforation of the abdominal wall can occur during colonoscopy, but this is a rare occurrence when the exam is performed by a physician highly skilled in the technique. The test is usually reserved for those with suspicious symptoms and is not a routine screening device. Nonetheless, it is recommended for certain patients if they are at high risk of developing colorectal cancer.

During colonoscopy, the physician can remove benign or precancerous polyps, in a procedure called a polypectomy, but if they are large, it may be difficult to remove them through the wire loop (the snare) of the colonoscope. Large polyps may be malignant, as well as those that are attached directly to the intestinal wall at their base. If the physician has any reason to believe a malignancy might exist, he may recommend abdominal surgery to remove them and to afford him an opportunity to thoroughly inspect the colon and the surrounding area. A pathological examination of tissue obtained during this surgery will give a definitive diagnosis.

Cancers of the colon and rectum are most often treated by surgical removal of the diseased portion of the colon plus a wide margin of healthy tissue around it. This is called a *subtotal colectomy*. Lymph nodes that drain the area will also be removed so that the oncologist can examine them for signs of metastasis. If the cancer has spread to adjacent organs, such as the bladder or the uterus, these, too, may be removed.

It is not always possible to reconnect the ends of the intestines after removing the cancerous portion. This will be dependent upon such factors as location and size of the tumor. If rejoining is not possible, a *permanent colostomy* is performed. In this procedure, the surgeon creates a new opening through the abdomen, substituting for the rectum and permitting elimination of feces. A person with a colostomy has normal bowel functions, but the elimination method is different. Sometimes a temporary colostomy is performed so that the bowels can rest during the time required for healing. This operation will be reversed later, and the method of elimination will return to normal. If the entire colon and rectum are removed, the surgeon performs an *ileostomy*. Both this procedure and colostomy require a small pouch to be placed over the opening of the stoma (an artificial opening created after surgery), to receive bowel movements. Ostomies are discussed further in Chapter 10.

Sometimes radiation therapy is used before surgery to shrink the cancer; other times it is used as a follow-up, especially if the rectum has been removed. Radium needles may be implanted in the rectum to treat cancer of that area. Cryosurgery is sometimes used to treat small cancers of the rectum. Doctors also suggest chemotherapy for patients with colorectal cancer.

After surgery and/or radiation for colorectal cancer, a gastroenterologist and/or medical oncologist will follow up on the patient's progress.

CANCERS OF THE URINARY TRACT AND THE MALE REPRODUCTIVE ORGANS

Most of these cancers are relatively rare, except for prostate cancer, whose incidence in men is second only to that of lung cancer. Together, the urogenital cancers represent a significant portion of cancers in both men and women.

Cancer of the kidney. The kidneys are two bean-shaped organs, each about four inches long, located on either side of the spinal column. Blood passes through the kidneys, which remove and dissolve the impurities, forming urine.

Cancer of the kidney is among the rarest forms of cancer; the types that develop in adults are usually referred to collectively as *renal-cell cancer*, or *hypernephroma*. (The fifth type of kidney cancer, called *Wilm's tumor*, develops only in children; it is successfully treated with surgery, radiation therapy, and chemotherapy.)

Adult kidney cancer is more common in men than in women, usually occurring between ages fifty and seventy. Some, but not all, kidney cancers develop in tobacco users.

The symptoms of kidney cancer are much like those of far less serious diseases. They include:

- Visible blood in the urine.
- A lump in the abdomen.
- Pain in the side.

and sometimes, the development of:

- Hypertension (high blood pressure).
- Low-grade fever, weight loss, and anemia.

The diagnostic procedure begins with a medical examination by a physician, followed by blood tests and urinalysis. An IVP, tomograms, and ultrasound can reveal if a suspected mass is a cyst or a tumor. A CAT scan and renal angiogram will yield additional information. Generally, these tests can determine whether a tumor is benign or malignant, but sometimes a biopsy is required. Occasionally, urologists perform a needle biopsy on the kidney. If the doctor strongly suspects or knows that you have cancer, further tests will be done to see if it has metastasized.

Treatment usually consists of surgery. *Simple nephrectomy* entails removing only the affected kidney. *Radical nephrectomy* includes removal of the kidney and large portions of the surrounding tissue together with the adjacent lymph nodes. Neighboring organs, if affected, may also have to be removed. The remaining kidney assumes the functions that were formerly shared by both.

Embolization (introduction of various substances to cut off the blood supply to the kidneys) at the time of the angiogram is sometimes used to shrink the tumor prior to surgery. Radiotherapy may be administered after surgery. Chemotherapy also may be used.

A urologist will perform the surgery, and you may also be followed up on by an internist and a medical oncologist.

Cancer of the bladder. The bladder is a muscular, elastic sac that stores urine before it is excreted from the body. It is located in the lower abdomen. The urine is carried down from each of the two kidneys to the bladder by long narrow tubes called ureters. The urine empties from the bladder through a muscular canal called the urethra. A woman's urethra is short; a man's is much longer, extending from the bladder past the prostate gland and through the penis.

Most tumors that begin in the bladder are called *papillary* tumors. They are shaped like small mushrooms with stems and are attached to the inner lining of the bladder. These cancerous papillomas tend to recur; for this reason, patients require continuous monitoring once they have developed even one. These tumors, which can invade underlying muscles of the bladder wall, are called *transitional-cell carcinomas*, and are a more advanced form of the previously described papillomas. This kind of cancer most often develops in people who work with certain aniline dyes, rubber, leather, print, paint, petroleum, and other industrial organic chemicals. Cigarette-smoking also is closely linked with bladder cancer, and saccharin is suspected as well. A history of chronic bladder infections may predispose a person to bladder cancer. Squamous-cell carcinomas are often either associated with or distinct from transitional-cell cancers.

The symptoms of bladder cancer are like symptoms of some other conditions, many of which are not malignant. They include:

- Constant or intermittent painless hematuria (blood in the urine), either visible or detectable only under a microscope.
- Fever.
- Frequent urination.
- Inability to urinate.
- Hesitancy, difficulty, or pain on urination.

The chief symptom is blood in the urine. Although that can be a symptom of many other problems, it should *never* be ignored, even if it is intermittent or stops.

If your physician suspects that you have bladder cancer (or any other urological problem), he will send you to a urologist, who will determine, by means of cytological examination, if cancer cells are present in your urine. He will examine the bladder contents by means of a cystoscopy and an intravenous pyelogram, and will perform other diagnostic tests and X rays to see if the disease has spread.

Small papillaries can be removed during cystoscopy by way of cauterization or electrodessication. This procedure, during which single or multiple small tumors can be removed, is usually done in the hospital, but it can be done on an outpatient basis. It is often described as a transurethral resection of the bladder tumor (TURBT). The cystoscope is passed from the opening of the urethra directly up into the bladder. If it is discovered during a TURBT that a tumor has invaded the bladder wall, open surgery may be required.

If only a part of the bladder is removed, urination will remain normal afterward. If the entire bladder is removed—in a procedure called a total cystectomy—an artificial bladder must be created to store urine. In one procedure, called a *urostomy*, the ureters are disconnected from the bladder and are joined to the end of a small segment of the ileum (part of the small intestine). This segment of the ileum is converted into a conduit, or tube, and is brought through the wall of the abdomen, near the navel, where it forms an opening called a stoma. This enables urine to flow out of the body. An appliance, often referred to as a flat bag or pouch, is placed over the stoma to collect urine. In Chapter 10 I will discuss living with a urostomy. (A recent medical advance is the creation of an artificial bladder, which does not require an external appliance.)

If the cancer has spread into adjacent organs, they, too, may also be removed. In men, the prostate, seminal vesicles, and ureter are routinely removed during the procedure. In women, the organs removed may include the ovaries, fallopian tubes, and/or uterus.

Recent advances have permitted some forms of bladder cancer that previously required surgical removal to be treated with chemotherapy, administered directly into the bladder. Standard chemotherapy and radiation are also used to treat bladder cancer.

Your urologist and a medical oncologist will monitor your progress after treatment.

Cancer of the prostate The prostate is an exclusively male gland that surrounds the urethra. It is located next to the inner wall of the rectum directly below the bladder, and secretes fluid that forms a part of semen.

As men age, the prostate tends to enlarge, in a condition that eventually affects most men, called *benign prostatic hypertrophy (BPH)*, which can interfere with urination. This is not a cancerous condition but often requires surgery to correct.

Cancer of the prostate is so common that, according to reliable estimates, by age eighty almost all men have had at least the early stages of it. Even if the cancer is untreated, or treated very conservatively but carefully watched, most of these elderly men will never show symptoms of cancer and will die of unrelated causes.

However, from age fifty-five to seventy-four, prostatic cancer is a very common cancer in men and, as I said earlier, is exceeded in numbers only by lung cancer. In these men, the disease *must* be treated. No definite causes have been identified for prostatic cancer, although some studies have shown that among men with low-cholesterol diets, as well as those who are vegetarians or eat a great many green and yellow vegetables, there is a lower-than-average incidence.

Prostate cancer can often be detected before the symptoms are noticeable and at a time when the cure rate is high. A digital rectal examination performed during a yearly (twice yearly for those over sixty) medical examination can identify any hard nodules in the prostate that may be cancerous. A family physician who finds such a nodule will generally send the patient to a urologist for further examination. Sometimes a man who has a benign condition that requires surgery will *also* have a malignancy, which will be discovered when tissue is examined by the pathologist. Although many men ask, it is not possible to examine your own prostate.

The signs and symptoms of prostate cancer are the same as those of benign prostatic hypertrophy, and no man should ignore them. They include:

- Weak or interrupted flow of urine.
- Unusually frequent urination.
- Inability or difficulty in beginning to urinate.

- Pain or burning during urination.
- Blood in urine.
- Pain in back, hips, or pelvis (even if unaccompanied by urinary problems).

If you notice any of these symptoms, you should go to your doctor, who will send you to a urologist to establish if cancer is present. Tests include specific blood tests, an intravenous pyelogram, and a cystoscope if warranted. Some urologists do a biopsy, in which a needle is inserted either into the patient's rectum, or between the scrotum and rectum. Tissue is then aspirated from the prostate. Since prostate cancer, like other cancers, has a tendency to metastasize, various scans and other tests that visualize the body will also be done, all prior to treatment.

Treatment varies according to the patient's age, extent of the disease, and other health factors. Different urologists and medical centers recommend different treatments for the same stage of prostate cancer, and it is wise to get more than one opinion, since the patient may ultimately wish to make a choice among offered treatments.

Surgery for prostatic obstruction from benign growth may include a procedure called *transurethral resection of the prostate (TUR or TURP)*, by means of which a surgeon can remove the prostatic tissue and relieve any urinary symptoms. During this procedure, an instrument is inserted into the penis and through the urethra (in the same manner as a cystoscope). It is often referred to as a "closed operation." Tissue removed during this procedure will be examined by the pathologist to determine if it is indeed benign; sometimes it is found to reveal an early cancer.

Other surgical procedures require an incision through the skin in the lower abdomen. The prostate itself, with or without the capsule in which it is enclosed, is subsequently removed. The seminal vesicles may also be removed. At one time, impotence and incontinence (inability to hold urine) were frequent side effects of such surgery, but recent advances in this technique have increasingly permitted preservation of potency and continence.

Radiotherapy is often the primary treatment for prostate cancer; it may be given externally, or a radioactive implant may be inserted into the prostate.

Because prostate cancer is dependent on male hormones for growth, another important treatment is to remove the supply of male hormones and/or to administer female hormones. Such treatment may be carried out through surgery, in a procedure called *orchidectomy* (or orchiectomy), the removal of the testicles, which are the source of male hormones. The scrotum remains, and a synthetic testicle can be implanted in it. This procedure is usually reserved for metastatic cancers.

Small doses of oral stilbestrol (a synthetic form of estrogen, a female hormone) may also be given to offset the male hormones, in addition to, or instead of, surgery. Other treatments include cryosurgery or laser surgery. Chemotherapy may also be offered.

It is important to note that despite advances in techniques, treatments for prostatic cancer can interfere with sexual functioning and cause impotence. During some procedures certain nerves may be destroyed. And depriving a man of his full supply of male hormones can lead to impotence and/or decreased sexual desire.

However, the female hormones do not radically "feminize" a man. His voice will not become high-pitched; and although his beard growth may lighten and his body shape may alter slightly, in general these changes are hardly noticeable to anyone but the patient himself.

A urologist performs surgery for prostatic cancer, and many urologists will follow up on the care of the patient. He may also be monitored by a medical oncologist.

Testicular cancer. The testicles, or testes, are the two male reproductive glands that produce sperm and androgens (male hormones). These oval organs, suspended behind the penis, are enclosed in the scrotum, a pouch of skin. A man with only one testicle remains sexually potent and is able to produce sperm.

There are approximately five thousand new cases of testicular cancer diagnosed in the United States each year. Most occur in young white men between the ages of twenty-five and forty. Usually only one testis is affected.

Those at very high risk are men who have a history of a testicle that was not descended from the abdomen. Men who have had a testicle surgically brought down into the scrotum, rather than removed, are also thought by some experts to be at risk. Others at risk (but far lower) are men whose fathers or brothers have had testicular cancer.

Some studies have suggested that young men whose mothers took diethylstilbestrol and other DES-type drugs during the time they were pregnant with them sometimes have small or undescended testicles. At this time there is no scientific evidence that DES in itself has caused an increased risk of testicular cancer in such men.

The first symptoms of testicular cancer are:

- A painless lump or swelling in a testicle.
- Dull ache in lower abdomen, groin, or scrotum.
- Feeling of heaviness in the scrotum.
- Breast enlargement (occurs because testicular cancer can cause a hormonal imbalance).

- Loss of sexual potency or sex drive.
- An occasional sharp pain in a testicle.

Painless enlargement is usually the first symptom and may occur when the cancer is still early. All men—young ones in particular—should be urged to regularly inspect their testicles, much as women are encouraged to do breast self-examination. Any changes should be reported immediately to a physician.

If the physician suspects testicular cancer (some benign conditions may have the same symptoms), he will send the patient to a urologist, who will recommend surgical exploration of the affected testicle. The testicle is explored through the groin, rather than just biopsied through the scrotum, because once the scrotum is opened, there is a risk of altering lymph-node drainage and thus complicating the disease (if cancer exists) and its treatment. The surgery is always scheduled as "exploration with possible removal."

Remember: The removal of one testicle does not preclude sexual activity, but some surgical procedures used to treat metastasized testicular cancer may lead to the inability to ejaculate, thus rendering a man sterile.

After the testicle is removed, it will then be thoroughly examined by the pathologist. There are two broad types of testicular cancers, *seminomas* and *nonseminomas*. They differ in the rate and route of spread and their response to treatment, so it is necessary to identify the type before treatment begins. In many instances, a synthetic testicle is implanted in the scrotum so that the man will look cosmetically the same as before.

Prior to surgery, or sometimes following it, several tests will be ordered to determine the extent of the cancer. A blood test can identify certain proteins in the bloodstream that are produced by testicular cancers. Two such proteins are called alpha-fetoprotein (AFP) and human chorionic gonadotropin (HCG), both helpful in determining the stage of testicular cancers and, later, in monitoring response to surgery and other treatments. Tests will be done to see if the lungs, liver, or bones have been affected, and a number of blood tests will reveal other information. An especially important test often utilized is the *lymphangiogram*, which will tell if the lymph nodes along the abdomen are involved. Certain types of testicular cancer warrant a lymph-node dissection. This separate procedure is lengthy and complicated but absolutely essential.

Treatment for testicular cancer has improved tremendously in recent years, and many men are completely cured who only a short time ago would have done very poorly. Testicular cancer is still fairly rare, and a patient should make sure that treatment is given by a team of physicians who are very experienced in the latest diagnostic procedures and treatments. Surgery, radiation, and chemotherapy may all be used in various sequences. A urologist and medical oncologist will probably be the patient's primary physicians.

Cancer of the penis. The penis, which is the male organ that serves for the discharge of urine and for sexual intercourse, is seldom the site of primary cancer. This cancer is extremely rare, particularly in the United States, and is confined almost exclusively to men between the ages of fifty and seventy. It has long been noted that cancer of the penis is most common in uncircumcised males; recent evidence indicates that obese circumcised men with poor hygiene are possibly at greater risk than uncircumcised men with good hygiene.

For many years it was thought that there was a relationship between cancer of the penis in men and cancer of the cervix in their female sexual partners. This theory is now obsolete.

When cancer of the penis occurs, it usually begins as a sore, wart, or ulcer at the end of the penis. Bleeding, discharge, and a lump in the groin are also symptoms of penis cancer.

Diagnosis is usually made by biopsy performed under local anesthesia. Treatment is usually the surgical removal of the lesion and sometimes a part of the penis, in a procedure called a *partial penectomy*. Occasionally it is necessary to surgically remove all of the penis. If the cancer has spread to the lymph glands, they, too, will be treated by surgery. Radiation and chemotherapy are also sometimes used.

A urologist will diagnose and treat cancer of the penis, sometimes in collaboration with a medical oncologist.

CANCERS OF THE FEMALE REPRODUCTIVE SYSTEM

Cancer of the uterus accounts for about 12 percent of all new cancers in women each year, ovarian cancer for 4 percent, and the other cancers of the female reproductive system (including in-situ carcinomas of the cervical uterus described later) bring the total to almost 25 percent.

The cancers of the female reproductive system include those of the uterus (cervix, endometrium, and placenta), ovaries, vulva, vagina, and fallopian tubes. As with many other cancers, when they are diagnosed early, the cure rate is high; advanced cancers have a less favorable outcome.

Cancer of the cervix. The cervix is the necklike portion of the uterus, or womb, that projects into the top of the vagina. Cancer of the cervix is very slow-growing; abnormal or premalignant cells may take any-where from three to twenty years before they are fully malignant and likely to metastasize to neighboring organs. For this reason, cervical cancer has an almost 100 percent cure rate when detected and treated early. As the cancer is allowed to progress, the cure rate diminishes.

Although cancer of the cervix occurs most frequently in women over thirty-five, women as young as age twenty can develop it. The exact cause of cervical cancer is unknown, but certain women are con-sidered at special risk. They are:

- Women who began having sexual intercourse before age eigh-teen.
- Women who have had multiple male sexual partners.
- Women with lower-than-average income.

It is possible, but not established, that women who have had herpes simplex II genital virus may also be at greater risk. Other recent re-search indicates that another type of virus, a papillomavirus, may also play a role in the eventual development of cancer of the cervix. This virus is associated with flat genital warts, known as condylomas. Some studies suggest that women who have had more than five children may also be at risk.

Women who have never had children, and those on menopausal estrogen-replacement therapy, have a lower-than-average risk. It is rare in women who have never had sexual intercourse.

There is one group of women who may, at any age, be at risk for a certain type of cervical cancer (as well as a rare vaginal cancer, de-scribed later). These are women whose mothers took diethylstilbestrol (DES), or some similar drugs, during the time they were pregnant with them. DES daughters, as these women are called, often have certain unusual tissue formations in the vagina and cervix. Approximately 250 young women out of the 1 to 2 million who were exposed to the drug while still in their mother's uterus have developed this unusual cancer in their teens or twenties; it remains to be seen whether other DES daughters will develop a related cancer at a later age. For this reason, and because these young women frequently have problems relating to menstruation and fertility, they are urged to have regular gynecological examinations beginning in their teens, and to inform their physician that their mother took this drug.

Cancer of the cervix is also referred to as *uterine cervical cancer* because the cervix is a part of the uterus. It can be detected in its earliest stage through periodic pelvic examinations, including Pap (short for Papanicolaou) smears. The American Cancer Society recommends that after two negative Pap smears one year apart women can wait three years before their next one. Many gynecological experts believe that a pelvic examination and the Pap test should be repeated yearly for *all* sexually active women since it is a painless, risk-free, and relatively inexpensive test.

An abnormal result to a Pap test alerts the physician to a condition called dysplasia, the presence of abnormal cells. Cervical dysplasia may be classified as mild, moderate, or severe, and in some women it will go through a series of changes, developing into cancer if it is not treated. Dysplasia has no symptoms; it is most often found in women between the ages of twenty-five and thirty-five, but it can occur earlier or later.

Carcinoma in situ is a term used to describe very early cancer. In this instance it refers to the growth of cancer cells on the top layer of the cervix, a condition that develops most often in women between the ages of thirty and forty, though sometimes earlier. It, too, is detected during the pelvic examination and Pap smear. It is curable in almost every case if treatment is started before the cancer has invaded the deeper layers of the cervix. Carcinoma in situ seldom causes any noticeable symptoms.

Invasive cancer of the cervix is just as it sounds: cancer that has grown deeper into the cervix. There may be no obvious symptoms, but if they do exist, they will probably include:

- Bleeding from the vagina—between regular menstrual periods, after sexual intercourse, or after a gynecological examination.
- Increased vaginal discharge.

Diagnosis of any of these cervical lesions begins with detection through the gynecological examination and the Pap test. A gynecological, or pelvic, exam includes examination of the external genitals, as well as of the vagina and cervix. The doctor will conduct a digital examination of both the vagina and the rectum; he will insert an instrument called a speculum into the vagina to widen it so that the interior may be more easily visible, and then collect a sample of cells for the Pap smear. The test results are classified in five ways:

Class 1: No abnormal cells (called a negative result).
Class 2: Inflammation or atypia (borderline cells but not cancerous).
Class 3: Dysplasia, suggestive of, or suspicious of, malignancy.
Class 4: Strongly suggestive of malignancy.
Class 5: Cancer cells definitely present.

If the result is Class 2 or higher, the gynecologist may repeat the Pap smear, then order further tests, perhaps including further biopsy (in or out of the hospital) to establish if indeed there is cancer, and if so, to determine the stage. One test is a *colposcopy* of the cervix, a technique of viewing the cervix through a magnifying instrument. Another test requires *conization*, a procedure in which a cone-shaped piece of tissue is removed from the cervix and cervical canal. Conization requires anesthesia and is done in the hospital.

For complete staging of cervical cancer, the physician will conduct a thorough pelvic exam and biopsy under general anesthesia. He may also perform an examination of the colon and rectum by sigmoidoscopy and GI series; a cystoscope and IVP of the bladder and ureters; and a lymphangiogram to visualize the lymph nodes.

Treatment of cervical cancer will depend on the extent of the disease. Dysplasia (which is *not* cancer) is sometimes left untreated but is carefully watched and usually treated with cryosurgery or cauterization. Severe dysplasia may be treated with conization. Laser surgery is sometimes employed.

Carcinoma in situ is usually treated with conization and careful follow-up by examination, repeat Pap smears and colposcopies in young women who still plan to have children. Doctors often recommend a hysterectomy to women who are certain they will not want to have children in the future. Hysterectomy, the surgical removal of the entire uterus, may be performed through the vagina or through an incision in the abdomen.

More-invasive cervical cancers may be treated by a radical hysterectomy: removal of the uterus, cervix, upper vagina, some surrounding tissue, and the lymph nodes in the area. If the malignancy has spread to adjacent organs, such as the bladder or rectum, these, too, may have to be removed.

Radiotherapy plays a major role in the treatment of cervical cancer. As discussed in Chapter 5, implants of radioactive substances are often used to treat cervical cancer. External radiation is also useful. Radiation may be offered in addition to or instead of surgery. Chemotherapy may be recommended as well.

A gynecologist is the primary physician for patients with cancer of the cervix, but other surgeons may also be involved. You may also be closely followed by a radiotherapist and medical oncologist.

Endometrial and uterine cancers. Cancer of the upper part of the uterus almost always begins in the endometrium, the mucous membrane that lines the interior of the uterus. Uterine cancer and endometrial cancer are terms used to refer to the same disease. This cancer most often occurs at around age fifty or sixty, often around the time when a woman stops having regular menstrual periods.

At high risk for the development of endometrial cancer are women who:

• have a medical history of infertility.
• have a medical history of irregular periods.

- have never been pregnant.
- were late in reaching menopause.
- are obese.
- suffer from diabetes.
- suffer from hypertension.
- have undergone prolonged estrogen-replacement therapy to relieve certain symptoms of menopause.
- have a tendency toward endometrial hyperplasia (increase in the number of cells in the endometrium).

The present or past use of the Pill, containing both estrogen and progesterone, does *not* pose a risk factor; instead, it appears to offer some (but not full) protection against the later development of endometrial cancer.

Regardless of any of the above factors, any woman who experiences the following symptoms should be examined for the possibility of cancer:

- Watery, blood-streaked discharge.
- Bleeding after menopause.
- Bleeding between periods.
- Lower-abdominal and lower-back pain.

It should be noted that several benign conditions can cause the same symptoms, so although a woman should call them to a doctor's attention, she shouldn't panic! The Pap smear, so accurate in detecting early cervical cancer, is not useful in detecting endometrial cancer; less than half the patients with this disease show positive test results. Based on his pelvic-examination findings and/or your reported symptoms, your gynecologist may suggest a curettage to extract endometrial cells from the uterus. This procedure is done in the office and is called an aspiration, vabra, vacuum, or suction, curettage. While it is an extremely uncomfortable procedure, most women find it tolerable. A few report it to be quite painful, so some doctors suggest a sedative prior to the procedure. There can be some severe cramping shortly afterward, so a woman is usually advised to have someone accompany her home, especially if she is driving. Most women find they can go about their normal routine the following day.

In addition to, or instead of, a vacuum curettage, the gynecologist may recommend a fractional D & C (dilatation and curettage) under general anesthesia. The cervix is expanded enough (dilated) to permit insertion of a small instrument that removes material from the uterine lining (curettage). This material is then sent to a pathologist for biopsy. The procedure is done in the hospital, and does not necessitate an overnight stay unless there is a medical reason for remaining.

In addition to the biopsy, other tests will be performed to determine if the cancer has spread beyond the uterus to other areas of the pelvis, or even to the bladder or rectum or beyond. In addition to blood tests and a chest X ray, the doctor may schedule an IVP, sigmoidoscopy and cystoscopy, scans, and a lymphangiogram.

Treatment usually involves surgery: hysterectomy (removal of the uterus) or a procedure called a *bilateral salpingo-oophorectomy*, removal of the ovaries and fallopian tubes as well as the uterus. Lymph nodes in the pelvis may also be removed. Radiation is sometimes given externally or implanted prior to or following surgery. Chemotherapy, including hormone therapy, may also be given.

Ovarian cancer. The ovaries are the two female reproductive organs that produce the ova (eggs) and the female hormones estrogen and progesterone. The ovaries are flat, olive-shaped organs, each approximately one inch long. During each menstrual cycle, an egg (ovum) is discharged from one of the ovaries into one of the two fallopian tubes, which lead into the uterus. There, the ovum is either fertilized by a sperm (if the woman has had intercourse) or shed with the lining of the uterus in the process known as menstruation.

Definite causes of ovarian cancer have yet to be identified, but some studies indicate that women at highest risk may be those who:

- are over forty years of age (or, more likely, past menopause).
- maintain a diet high in animal fat, low in vegetable fat and fiber.
- use talcum powder (sometimes contaminated with particles of asbestos) in genital area or on diaphragms.
- have a close-family (mother or sister) history of ovarian cancer.
- have a history of ovarian problems (imbalance or malfunction).
- have a history of breast cancer.
- have undergone estrogen-replacement therapy after menopause. (This risk factor is still inconclusive).
- have never had children.

The less a woman has ovulated in her lifetime, the *lower* her risk of ovarian cancer; thus, women who have taken birth-control pills seem to have a lower risk of developing this disease in later years; those who have had several children and/or first child prior to age twenty-two may also be in a low-risk bracket. These are statistical findings, but as yet no conclusive explanations have been offered.

Early detection of ovarian cancer seems to be impossible. No tests available today can show the beginnings of the disease, although a gynecologist is always suspicious of enlarged ovaries in postmenopausal women and may seek a diagnostic workup.

Symptoms indicative of ovarian cancer are often vague and tend to be ignored by patient and doctor alike. They are:

- Persistent indigestion, gassiness, belching, or heartburn.
- Feelings of fullness after eating only a small amount of food.
- Expansion of waistline or stomach, not due to "usual" reasons of weight gain.

Women often report these symptoms to a family physician or gastroenterologist, rather than their gynecologist. However, any physician who suspects ovarian cancer will quickly refer her to a gynecologist, who will conduct a pelvic examination. If he finds an enlarged ovary, he will order tests including (but not necessarily in this order) chest X rays, an IVP, lower GI series, various scans, ultrasound, a lymphangiogram (this may wait until after diagnosis), and possibly a biopsy with a laparoscope. During a *laparoscopy*, a small incision is made in the abdomen. A lighted tube is then inserted, allowing the doctor to examine the ovaries and abdominal interior and to remove a piece of tissue for biopsy. Some gynecologists reserve laparoscopy for young patients with enlarged ovaries; in older patients, or when ovarian cancer is strongly suspected (or if other tests fail to distinguish between a cyst and a malignant tumor), a *laparotomy* is performed. In this surgical procedure, the doctor makes an incision through the wall of the abdomen to inspect the ovaries and abdominal interior. Tissue is removed for biopsy, and a frozen section (see page 25) can be performed.

Ovarian cancer is treated by surgical removal of both ovaries and sufficient adjacent structures and tissues (often including the uterus and fallopian tubes) to eliminate as much of the tumor as possible and to accurately stage the disease. Although any competent gynecologist can perform this surgery, many experts believe it should only be done by one who is very experienced in treating ovarian cancer. Thus, even if ovarian cancer is only *suspected*, a patient should be sure she has chosen a gynecologist with that experience.

Most of the information necessary to stage ovarian cancer is obtained during the laparotomy. The type of cell in which the tumor began is identified, as well as the grade and stage. Cells in a high-grade tumor have few normal characteristics; cells in a low-grade tumor have many normal characteristics. The earliest (lowest) stage is limited to disease involving only one ovary with no ascites (abnormal fluid in the abdominal cavity); later (higher) stages may include disease in both ovaries, bowels, liver, and outside the abdominal cavity. The type, grade, and stage of the disease will determine treatment.

Unfortunately, ovarian cancer is usually not diagnosed until it has grown beyond the earliest stage, necessitating aggressive treatment. Thus, following surgery, most ovarian-cancer patients will require chemotherapy and possibly radiotherapy. Some of the newer, more powerful drugs, such as platinum, have significantly improved the ovarian-cancer patient's survival rate.

Just as this disease is difficult to detect in the early stage, so is it also difficult to measure the response to treatment. Therefore, after a specific course of chemotherapy has been completed (usually one to two years), a "second look"—abdominal surgery—is necessary. If cancer is still present, treatment will be continued or changed. If there is no sign of disease, treatment may be stopped, but the patient is carefully observed. Sometimes a "third look" operation becomes necessary.

The ovarian-cancer patient will probably have two primary physicians: a gynecologist and a medical oncologist. Some patients choose to be monitored by one of the small number of gynecological oncologists who can give them total care, including any surgical procedures and chemotherapy.

Cancer of the vulva. The vulva are the external female genitals: the mons veneris, the labia majora, the labia minora, the vestibule of the vagina, and the vestibular glands. They are sometimes referred to as the "lips" of the vagina.

Cancer of the vulva is fairly rare and seldom develops before menopause. Symptoms may include burning, itching, bleeding, and discharge. Premalignant changes consisting of whitish, plaquelike lesions are very successfully treated by surgically removing the skin of the lips of the vulva and clitoris. More advanced cancer of the vulva may be treated with more extensive surgery, chemotherapy and/or internal or external radiation.

Cancer of the vagina. The vagina is the canal that leads from a woman's vulva to her cervix. It is located behind the bladder and in front of the rectum. It is also known as the birth canal.

Cancers of the vagina are rare, and until the late 1960s were found almost exclusively in women over fifty. However, at that time a number of young women with clear-cell vaginal cancer were identified. All of them had one thing in common: Their mothers had taken diethylstilbestrol (DES) or a related drug during the time they were pregnant with them. Although the total number of those who developed the cancer is small, compared to the total number of women exposed in utero to the drug, the incidence is significant enough that all DES daughters are considered at risk.

Symptoms of vaginal cancer include:

- Discharge, spotting, or bleeding—between periods; following intercourse or pelvic exam.

- Unusually frequent urination.
- Bladder discomfort or pain.

The National Cancer Institute recommends that *all* DES daughters, starting at either the time of their first menstrual period or age fourteen (whichever comes first), have yearly pelvic examinations and at least one colposcopy. If there is vaginal bleeding at a younger age than that, one is advised to see a physician at once. Women for whom vaginal cancer is suspected must also have a colposcopy.

Treatment depends on type, location, and stage of disease, as well as on the age of the patient. Surgery may include removal of the vagina (a new one can be reconstructed afterward), and further surgery if the disease has spread. Both internal and external radiation are used. Chemotherapy may be recommended.

Cancer of the fallopian tubes. The fallopian tubes are the passageways through which the ova move from the ovaries to the uterus. Cancer of the fallopian tubes is extremely rare, and when it does occur, it is usually (but not always) in women between fifty and sixty. It can occur at other ages. Blood-tinged, honey-colored watery discharge or irregular vaginal bleeding may be symptoms. A positive Pap-smear result will lead to further investigation, including a D & C and ultrasound. Diagnosis is sometimes dependent upon surgical biopsy. Treatment will include a hysterectomy, and radiation and/or chemotherapy.

Choriocarcinoma. This cancer is a very rare tumor of the uterus that develops in the placenta of a pregnant woman. The placenta is the organ that forms during pregnancy and through which the fetus absorbs oxygen, nutrients, and other substances, and excretes wastes.

Women who develop choriocarcinoma frequently (but not necessarily) have had one or more of the following:

- An ectopic pregnancy (a pregnancy that takes place in the fallopian tubes rather than the uterus and must be terminated).
- A molar pregnancy (in which signs of pregnancy are all exaggerated including abnormal growth of uterus).
- An abortion, and a pregnancy blood test that is positive long after the pregnancy is terminated.

It is a very fast-growing cancer, and its first symptoms are often a repeated and chronic cough or trouble breathing, because the choriocarcinoma spreads quickly to the lungs. At one time the disease was always fatal, but today, with chemotherapy, it is highly curable. Choriocarcinoma should be treated at a medical center or by a physician, usually a medical oncologist, who is very familiar with the disease.

A gynecologist is the primary physician for all cancers of the female reproductive system, but you may also be followed up on closely by a medical oncologist. As we discussed on pages 000–000, there are gynecologists who specialize in treating cancers of the reproductive system. You may wish to see a gynecological oncologist for a second opinion prior to surgery, even if you prefer your own gynecologist to take care of you.

CANCER OF THE BRAIN AND SPINAL CORD

The brain is the portion of the central nervous system enclosed within the skull. The brain's nerve tissue extends to the spinal cord, which is the network of nerve tissue extending through the spinal canal, the cavity within the vertebral column (better known as the backbone).

Brain tumors make up 2 to 5 percent of all cancers and most often occur in men and women between the ages of forty and sixty. Young children and teenagers may also develop brain tumors.

Unlike other cancers, malignant brain tumors do not metastasize. But they are resistant to total destruction by means of surgery, radiation, or chemotherapy—and they tend to recur.

Almost half of all brain tumors are benign, but they must be carefully watched or treated, because they can cause life-threatening symptoms. They are far more easily cured or controlled for long periods of time than are malignant ones.

Generally, primary brain tumors (those that originate in the brain) can be divided into these types:

Gliomas are the most common type of malignant brain tumor, originating within the brain tissue. There are several types of gliomas, and various grades of each type. The higher the grade of the tumor, the faster it grows.

Medulloblastomas are malignant brain tumors that develop in young children. They arise in the cerebellum and, without treatment, spread rapidly into the spinal fluid and to other parts of the brain and spinal cord.

Meningiomas are usually benign. These tumors begin in the tissue membranes and tend to grow large.

Neuromas are benign, slow-growing tumors that originate in the nerves, occurring mostly in people over forty.

Symptoms are reflective of the exact location and type of tumor. They may include:

- A seizure.
- Severe or persistent headaches.
- Increasing irritability.
- Personality changes.
- Unusual fatigue or sleeplessness.
- Nausea and vomiting.
- Difficulties with hearing, visual speech, taste, smell, or balance.

Often these symptoms are initially attributed to something less serious, and hence ignored; only a seizure will alarm the patient or his family.

Tumors that begin in the spinal cord may affect the nerves between the brain and the body in much the same way as an accident to the spinal cord. Pain, loss of feeling, or mild to complete paralysis may occur.

Diagnosis is accomplished through a history of symptoms and a medical examination of the eyes, muscle functions, reflexes, and ability to feel pinpricks. A spinal tap, skull X rays, CAT scans, EEG, angiograms, sonograms, and other tests that can visualize the brain will probably be ordered. A small tissue biopsy may be taken for examination.

A neurosurgeon may surgically remove part or all of a tumor in the brain or on the spinal cord; often the patient will receive radiotherapy and chemotherapy. Some new drugs are able to penetrate the "blood-brain barrier," a mechanism that generally prevents most substances in the bloodstream from entering the brain. Steroids are usually prescribed to prevent swelling in the brain and to relieve symptoms.

Care of the patient with cancer of the brain or central nervous system will usually be managed by a neurologist (a medical doctor who treats diseases of the brain and nervous system), a neurosurgeon, and/or a medical oncologist.

CANCERS OF THE BONE

Bones are the dense, hard, and slightly elastic connective tissue that make up most of the skeletal system. They form a rigid framework that bears body weight, provides fixed points for muscle action, and protects vital organs. Other tissues, such as blood vessels, cartilage, and bone marrow, are closely related to—and affected by—the skeletal system.

Tumors can arise in any of these tissues. Cancers that arise in bones and from tissues that connect or lie between organs and skin are referred to as *sarcomas*.

There are two classifications of sarcomas: bone cancers, which begin in the hard substance of bones; and soft-tissue sarcomas, which start in muscle, fat, fibrous tissue, blood vessels, nerves, or other supporting tissue of the body. Most bone cancers are sarcomas, but those that arise in the bone marrow and other blood-forming tissues are classified as *lymphomas*.

Sarcomas are relatively rare: Approximately 1,900 new cases of bone cancer are diagnosed each year, and approximately 4,900 new cases of soft-tissue sarcoma. Together they account for less than 2 percent of all new cancer cases each year.

Many cancers that begin in other areas of the body metastasize to the bones, forming secondary tumors there.

Despite the differences in types of bone cancer, they share one common symptom: pain. A persistent ache may be a sign of bone cancer; the knee, thigh, upper arm, ribs, and pelvis are the most common sites. Swelling or fever may accompany the pain.

Types of Bone Cancers

Osteogenic sarcoma, more common during childhood and adolescence than during adulthood, often begins with a tumor in the bones in a leg or arm. Surgical removal of the tumor is usually the method of treatment, preceded or followed by chemotherapy. Amputation of the affected limb was once the traditional treatment to prevent recurrence and spreading of the cancer. Today, however, chemotherapy has made it possible for doctors to avoid amputation in many cases.

Ewings's sarcoma, a fast-growing cancer, begins in the marrow spaces inside the midshafts of bones. Chemotherapy is an extremely effective treatment in this case; radiotherapy and surgery are also performed.

Chondrosarcoma occurs mostly in people of middle age but can also develop in children. It usually begins in the cartilage of a leg, hip, or rib, and it grows slowly. Surgery is the usual method of treatment, sometimes requiring amputation of the limb.

Fibrosarcoma arises in the ends of major limb bones and may spread into soft tissues. It occurs most often in middle-aged and elderly people and is treated by surgery, and sometimes radiation and chemotherapy as well.

Giant-cell tumor, a benign tumor that sometimes becomes cancerous, is more common in women than in men. The tumor is surgically removed along with a margin of tissue. In some malignant cases, amputation is necessary.

Chordoma is very rare. It occurs in the vertebrae, lower spinal column, or skull (where it can affect vision). It is usually treated with radiation.

Soft-tissue sarcomas, depending on the age of the patient and the exact location of the tumor, are most often treated with a combination of surgery, chemotherapy, and radiation.

Kaposi's sarcoma, historically a disease of elderly male patients, is a slow-growing cancer in which dark blue or purple-brown nodules occur on the skin or mucuous membranes. In 1981 a large outbreak of the disease was noted in much younger men, and ultimately it was seen to be related to an acutely suppressed immune system—in particular, acquired immune deficiency syndrome (AIDS). Most AIDS patients are homosexual men, but those who share hypodermic needles or who have been injected with contaminated blood are also at risk for the disease.

Most patients with bone cancers are treated by orthopedists who are experienced in treating these diseases. Patients are also followed by medical oncologists and/or radiotherapists.

SKIN CANCER

The skin is the body's protective covering. It is composed of two main layers: The surface layer is called the epidermis; the inner layer is the dermis.

Cancer of the skin is the most common of all cancers, accounting for over 400,000 new cases each year. It has been estimated that one out of every seven white people in the United States will eventually (usually in their later years) develop a skin cancer during their lifetime. When statistics for cancer are compiled, most of these are not even counted because they are the basal-cell or squamous-cell carcinomas, which together are 95 percent curable. Malignant melanoma, a far more serious form of skin cancer, requires prompt treatment and careful follow-up.

Anyone who spends a great deal of time in the sun is at risk of developing skin cancer, but those most at risk are those described as having "Celtic skin," such as those with fair skin and blue or green eyes.

Others at risk are people who have had exposure to radiation from X rays, chemicals such as coal tars and arsenic, thermal burns, and chronic draining sinus tracts.

This cancer may take years to develop, but most physicians now believe that everyone, especially those at risk, should avoid exposure to the ultraviolet light of the sun. Those people unwilling or unable to stay out of the sun should use the excellent sun screens and sun blocks that are now available in all drugstores. Some block the sun's harmful rays almost completely.

Symptoms of the various forms of skin cancer that should be brought to the attention of a dermatologist (a physician who specializes in diseases of the skin) include:

- Any unusual discoloration or change in an existing birthmark or mole.
- An existing or new sore that doesn't heal.
- A growth that continues to enlarge, itch, scab, or bleed.

Some lesions may be precancerous; these are called *actinic, solar,* or *senile, keratoses.* The dermatologist may decide to keep an eye on such lesions, waiting to treat them if and when they change, or he may remove them immediately, using topical chemotherapy, electrodesiccation, curettage, or cryosurgery. These lesions are then biopsied to establish a definitive diagnosis.

Basal-cell carcinomas. This is the most common type of skin cancer. Almost half of these carcinomas begin on the sun-exposed areas of the nose and cheeks, sometimes also near the eyes, or on the back or chest. They grow slowly, starting as small, painless, pale papules (smaller than nodules). The lesions may extend, eventually ulcerating and becoming covered with a scab or crust. Basal-cell carcinomas rarely metastasize, but if untreated, they can badly damage underlying tissues and structures, causing infections or hemorrhage. They can even directly invade a vital structure, such as the bones or the brain. Almost all—some estimates say 99 percent—of these cancers are cured completely, but in about 25 percent of cases, a new one will appear later, elsewhere on the skin. For this reason, people who have had a basal-cell carcinoma should carefully monitor their own skin and report any changes to a dermatologist.

Squamous-cell carcinomas. These skin cancers also tend to grow slowly, but unlike basal-cell carcinomas, they may metastasize to regional lymph nodes. They usually begin as a slightly raised pink opaque papule or patch, with irregular borders, later ulcerating in the center. These ulcerations increase in size as the cancer grows. Most of these cancers develop on the face, lips, backs of hands, rims of ears, and other sun-exposed areas.

These skin cancers are usually treated with outpatient or office procedures. Topical chemotherapy creams may be prescribed for some precancerous types. Other lesions are treated with cryosurgery, excisional surgery, electrosurgery, or chemosurgery (all of which are described in full on pages 37–39). Radiotherapy is also sometimes used, especially if the lesion is an area of cosmetic importance, or in elderly patients. Some dermatologists can treat these cancers with radiation in their own office; others send you to a radiotherapist. Occasionally, skin grafting or plastic-surgery repair is necessary when a large lesion has been removed.

A dermatologist treats basal-cell and squamous-cell carcinomas of the skin, and, if necessary, may send you to a plastic surgeon.

Malignant melanoma. This cancer is highly malignant, originating from a special cell called a melanocyte, which synthesizes melanin, the only pigment found in humans.

Melanomas can appear anywhere on the skin but most often begin on the trunk, head, neck, or arm in men; on the leg, arm, trunk, head, or neck in women.

Melanoma arises from an existing mole or as a new growth, beginning as a mottled dark patch, raised slightly above the skin, with irregular borders. The color may be mottled shades of tan or brown, intermingled with black, red, blue, and white. The surrounding skin may become red, swollen, and tender. It is often the size of a pencil eraser. Occasionally it ulcerates, becoming like an open sore that bleeds.

A person should have any pigmented moles in areas exposed to constant irritation (such as from clothing) removed, and should report any new skin patches or changes in moles to a dermatologist. If he has any suspicion, however mild, that you have a melanoma, rather than just a harmless mole, he will remove all or part of the growth himself (along with a wide margin of surrounding tissue) or send you to a general surgeon to have it done. A biopsy will then be performed on the removed tissue, to discover if the growth is a melanoma and, if it is, to stage the disease.

Malignant melanoma has a tendency to spread through the blood and lymph system to nearby lymph nodes, and can also metastasize to other organs. Thus, even a very small melanoma can be a serious life-threatening form of cancer and should not be viewed as "just a little skin cancer."

Some experts believe that all surgery for melanoma should be done by a dermatologist who has wide experience in treating this condition;

others believe that it should be done only by a general surgeon who is experienced in cancer surgery. Even if a dermatologist removes the melanoma, a general surgeon performs any further surgery, such as the removal of any nearby lymph nodes that are affected. Skin may have to be grafted from another part of the body to cover the surgical incision if it is very large or deep.

If the melanoma is at an early stage, surgery may be sufficient treatment. Where there has been some spread, chemotherapy—sometimes directly into the affected area—and immunotherapy, may be used. Radiation may be used as a palliative therapy.

Even where melanoma appears to be cured by early surgery, the patient should be closely monitored by a medical oncologist, who is best able to evaluate any changes that may indicate a recurrence of the disease. Unlike basal-cell and squamous-cell carcinomas, malignant melanoma is more likely to recur (if it does) as a metastatic disease rather than as another visible skin growth.

LEUKEMIA

Leukemia is a term that describes a variety of cancers of the blood or circulatory system in which abnormal white blood cells accumulate in the blood and bone marrow. The leukemic cells crowd the bone marrow, spill into circulating blood, and infiltrate such organs as the liver, lungs, and kidneys. They can even cross the blood-brain barrier, invading the brain and spinal cord.

The blood, as we have discussed earlier in the book, supplies nutrients, oxygen, hormones, and other chemicals to the body's cells. The blood transports these substances to the various organs of the body and also helps in the removal of waste products. Each blood component has a specific task, and some act as the body's defense against infection. Because the bone marrow does not maintain normal production in a person with leukemia, he is susceptible to fatigue, bleeding, and infection. His bone marrow will also contain more than the normal amount of blasts (immature cells), sending them into the bloodstream and causing an acute life-threatening condition.

There are several kinds of leukemia. The acute leukemias include acute lymphocytic leukemia (ALL) and acute nonlymphocytic leukemia (ANLL; sometimes referred to as acute myelocytic leukemia, or AML). Symptoms of the acute leukemias vary somewhat, as does their treatment. Chronic leukemias are collectively referred to as CML. Chronic myelocytic leukemia (also known as chronic granulocytic leukemia and chronic myelogenous leukemia) most commonly affects adults between the ages of thirty and sixty. Chronic lymphocytic leukemia (CLL) seldom begins before midlife; usually after fifty or sixty.

Together, the leukemias account for about 5 percent of all new cancer cases each year. Half of them are described as *acute,* the other half as *chronic.* More men than women develop the disease. Acute leukemia often affects children; ALL is the most common form.

The following factors are known to increase the risk of developing leukemia:

- Certain chromosomal abnormalities, such as Down's syndrome; and other genetic factors.
- Large doses of radiation (survivors of atomic-bomb explosions and radiologists who practiced in the early days of radiology are among high-risk individuals).
- Disorders of the immune system.
- Long-term exposure to certain chemicals that suppress bone-marrow function (e.g., benzene, aromatic hydrocarbon).
- Past treatment with certain chemotherapy drugs.
- Retroviruses (also known as RNA tumor viruses or type-C viruses).

The symptoms of the acute leukemias are not always readily apparent or recognized. They are:

- Lymph-node, spleen, and liver enlargement.
- Fever.
- Paleness.
- Loss of appetite.
- Fatigue.
- Frequent infections.
- Bone or joint pain.
- Tendency to bleed or bruise easily.

In children, for whom frequent mild illnesses are commonplace, the symptoms are usually no cause for alarm. They should, of course, be investigated if they persist, in either a child or an adult.

The symptoms of chronic leukemia are generally more subtle. Often the disease is not diagnosed until a person has a routine blood test. When symptoms appear, they may include:

- General feeling of fatigue, lack of energy.
- Fever.
- Loss of appetite.
- Night sweats.

- Enlarged lymph nodes in neck or groin.
- Heat intolerance.
- Easy bruising.

Diagnosis of the leukemias can often be made by a blood test that shows levels of hemoglobin, normal white blood cells, and platelets; and detects the presence of leukemic blast cells. The complete diagnosis is established with a bone-marrow biopsy. In this procedure, the physician inserts a long hollow needle into the chest or hip bone and suctions out a sample of the marrow. Sometimes several samples are taken. Laboratory analysis can distinguish between types of leukemia as well as determine extent of the disease. A spinal tap, in which fluid is removed from the spine, may also be done, to learn if the central nervous system has been affected.

The outlook for leukemia patients has improved greatly in recent years. Long-term remissions and cure are possible for patients who once had little hope.

Acute leukemias in both children and adult are usually treated with intensive chemotherapy, and radiation. Radiation is sometimes directed at the brain even if the leukemia cells have not affected it. This is called *central nervous system preventive therapy*, and it has helped to prevent relapses in some patients. Certain chemotherapy drugs that can penetrate the blood-brain barrier may also be used; some are administered directly into the spinal fluid.

A relatively new treatment is bone-marrow transplantation. It involves the transplant of bone marrow from a healthy, matched donor, usually a close relative. It is a complicated procedure, particularly for the recipient, and can only be done at some medical centers. (For further description, see pages 74–75.) Transfusions of matched blood platelets, and occasionally white blood cells, are also used occasionally.

Infections are difficult to control in leukemia patients, so sometimes during the course of treatment, if a patient seems at very high risk for infection, he may be placed in a relatively germ-free environment in the hospital. Anyone coming into his room must take special precautions (sterile gowns, masks, etc.) in a procedure called "reverse isolation." Sometimes a patient is placed in a sterile environment called a laminar air-flow room. These facilities are not available everywhere.

Chronic leukemia begins and progresses slowly. Often the patient is not treated immediately but is closely monitored. When treatment is given, it usually consists of chemotherapy and radiotherapy.

Interferon has been shown to be highly effective in patients with a rare type of leukemia *called hairy-cell leukemia*.

The leukemias are complicated diseases to treat. Patients may have remissions, during which they feel fine; then relapses, at which time acute symptoms reappear. Child and adult leukemia patients should be treated by a hematologist or medical oncologist who specializes in these diseases, and who can refer you to a medical center with the most sophisticated techniques (bone-marrow transplants, sterile laminar airflow rooms) if the need arises.

LYMPHOMAS

Lymphoma is a general term used to describe any cancer that develops in the lymphatic system. Lymph is a thin, milky-colored fluid that originates in many organs and tissues of the body and contains white blood cells. An important function of lymph is to bathe tissues and to aid in transportation of materials to the blood; it is sometimes referred to as the "second circulatory system." Lymphatic vessels are distributed throughout the body but are concentrated in regions around the neck, armpits, and upper chest; behind the ears; and inside the abdomen.

Lymphomas form in the lymphatic system, most commonly in the lymph nodes that are the small oval structures which act as sieves, filtering lymph and fighting infection. They also can arise in the spleen and lymph glands.

There are several types of cancers of the lymph system: One is called Hodgkin's disease; the others are collectively described as non-Hodgkin's lymphoma.

Hodgkin's disease develops in approximately ten thousand people each year. It is characterized by a painless progressive enlargement of the lymphoid tissue, usually beginning in the upper half of the body. Hodgkin's disease most often develops in young people between the ages of fifteen and thirty-four, or in others over the age of fifty.

At one time, patients with Hodgkin's disease had a very poor outlook, even if their disease was diagnosed at an early stage. Fortunately, that has now changed; 90 percent of those patients diagnosed in an early stage are cured with radiation alone. Even those who were diagnosed after the disease had progressed are doing well ten years after receiving treatment.

Non-Hodgkin's lymphomas, of which there are several kinds, resemble Hodgkin's disease, but a pathologist can see differences when he examines tissues under a microscope. These lymphomas often begin outside the lymph nodes and spread in a more disorderly fashion than Hodgkin's disease.

Although the following symptoms are also present in many less serious illnesses, particularly in young people, Hodgkin's disease or another lymphoma is often suspected when they are present.

- Painless swelling of lymph nodes, often in neck, sometimes in groin or armpit (referred to by some people as "swollen glands").
- Enlarged spleen.
- Fatigue.
- Pain in lymph nodes after drinking alcohol.
- Itching.
- Pain in abdomen, back, or legs.
- Nausea and vomiting.
- Weight loss.
- Fever.
- Night sweats.

When a patient reports these symptoms, his physician will conduct a thorough medical examination, taking particular notice if the spleen and lymph nodes are enlarged. He will conduct a number of blood tests and may then order various X rays, lymphangiograms, and scans. If these tests point to a likely diagnosis of a lymphoma, he will usually order a biopsy of a lymph node. The presence of certain cells called Reed-Sternberg cells and malignant reticulum cells establish the diagnosis of Hodgkin's disease. Patients with this disease sometimes undergo a laparotomy: abdominal surgery that makes it possible to precisely stage the disease. At the same time, the spleen is sometimes removed so that it can be examined for disease. This also avoids irradiation of the spleen that might damage adjacent organs.

When a diagnosis is firmly established and the disease has been staged, treatment begins. Hodgkin's patients, as I said earlier, are often completely cured with radiation therapy if the disease is limited in spread and symptoms are at a minimum. Those patients whose disease has spread and who have had several symptoms, such as weight loss and night sweats, will probably require chemotherapy as well.

Some lymphomas are slow-growing; others tend to spread quickly if not treated. Children often develop lymphomas, and many are treated successfully by surgery, chemotherapy, and radiation. Adult patients are often treated with radiation and/or chemotherapy.

Both Hodgkin's disease and the non-Hodgkin's lymphomas should be treated by a medical oncologist or hematologist along with a radiotherapist who is very experienced in treating these particular diseases.

MULTIPLE MYELOMA

Multiple myelomas are those cancers that form tumors composed of the plasma cells, normally found in the bone marrow. Myeloma may form simultaneously in the ribs, vertebrae, pelvic bones, and other sites. Patients with multiple myeloma are very vulnerable to infections because their plasma cells are not producing antibodies for their immune system to use against foreign invaders.

The disease is usually seen in people who are over fifty years old. Symptoms of multiple myeloma are:

- Severe and constant pain in back, ribs, neck, or pelvic areas.
- Anemia and fatigue.
- Bleeding gums, frequent nosebleeds, or other abnormal bleeding.
- Unexplained fractures or cracks of the bones.
- Painful swellings on ribs.
- Kidney problems.
- Weight loss.
- Recurrent bacterial infections.

When a patient reports these symptoms, his doctor will order a number of blood and urine tests, which in themselves may indicate the presence of the disease. A bone-marrow biopsy, and X rays and scans of the skeletal system can be used to confirm the diagnosis.

Treatment usually consists of chemotherapy and/or radiation and should be administered by a hematologist or medical oncologist.

This section has covered the most common types of cancer. If you wish to read further, several of the books listed in Appendix VII go into more detail. Your librarian can also help you find articles in magazines or journals for both the general public and the health professional.

The next section will deal with living through cancer. I will discuss the ways to best minimize and cope with the effects of treatment and pain, what to do about nutrition, and tell how many other health professionals can help you deal with cancer in yourself or someone you care about.

Section Four

LIVING THROUGH CANCER

Chapter 10

Minimizing and Coping with the Effects of Surgery

Radical surgery involving the removal of part or all of an organ may cause a change in the way you function, and you will need to make adaptations and adjustments. Surgery that alters a person's appearance (whether or not it is visible to others) can affect self-esteem and will require a period of adaptation and adjustment. Mastectomy, ostomies, amputations, any surgery to the head and neck, and orchidectomy (removal of testicles) are examples of surgical procedures that might be described as "trade-offs" for increasing survival from cancer.

Knowing what may occur and preparing for it can often minimize and help you cope with the sometimes traumatic effects of your treatment.

THE EFFECTS OF MASTECTOMY

The loss of a breast is seen by many women as a major loss to their concept of sexual self. Thousands of women have ignored the symptoms of breast cancer or, even when faced with it, refused surgery, because they did not want to lose a breast.

The possibility or reality of a mastectomy evokes a complex set of feelings. Women are naturally fearful and concerned about their survival from the cancer; at the same time they may be equally or more upset because of the loss of their breast. Many women feel as if their femininity has been diminished or even destroyed, and their self-image and self-esteem suffers. This is a common feeling and should never be dismissed as mere vanity. It often bears little relationship to age or whether a woman has, expects, or even wants a regular sexual partner.

A warm and caring husband or lover can do much to let a woman know she is "far more than just a breast." Women who have had mastectomies can often assure her that their marriages and relationships have not been threatened by the surgery, and others can tell of making new and lasting relationships after their mastectomy.

Physicians, nurses, and social workers can be very helpful to the woman faced with mastectomy. (Chapter 16 discusses the emotional reactions to cancer in more detail.)

Many women with breast cancer are now treated with alternative methods as described in Chapter 9, but others have no choice. The only way to halt the spread of their cancer is to have a mastectomy. Surgery today, as I said earlier, is not as radical as it once was, and with time, emotional support, and some rehabilitative exercises, a woman can generally return to her former activities.

Lymphedema

Following surgery, some women develop swelling in the arm on the side of the mastectomy. This may also occur following radiation for breast cancer if the treatment is directed to the lymph-node area. The condition is called *lymphedema*, the collection of excess fluid, and it is caused by the loss of, or damage to, the underarm lymph nodes and their connecting vessels. The circulation of the lymph fluid may be slowed, and the ability to fight infection may also be affected. It is considered a complication, rather than an expected side effect; special exercises and an elastic sleeve to stimulate circulation can often help.

Women who have either had lymph nodes removed or have been treated with radiation need to watch for lymphedema, and should also take special precautions to avoid infection.

Thus many physicians advise these patients:

- Be sure that all injections, vaccinations, blood samples, and blood-pressure tests are done on the other arm.
- Avoid carrying heavy packages or handbags on the affected side.
- Avoid cuts on hands and arms. Be careful with knives, gardening tools, and use a thimble when sewing. When you have a manicure, don't have your cuticles cut.
- If you shave under your arm, use an electric razor.
- If you do get a cut, wash it carefully and promptly, treat with antibacterial medication, and check often for signs of infection (soreness, redness).
- Avoid wearing tight jewelry, watches, and tight or elastic cuffs on the affected side.

- Use protective gloves when using any strong detergents.
- Avoid as many harsh and abrasive chemicals as possible.

If an infection should develop on the treated arm, or if the arm becomes painful, hot, red, or it swells, call your doctor at once. But don't "pamper" your arm unnecessarily or it can become dependent and useless.

Reach to Recovery

Reach to Recovery is a volunteer program sponsored by the American Cancer Society. It is based on the concept that a woman who has recovered from a mastectomy is able to offer emotional support and practical suggestions to another woman who has just had the same procedure. The Reach to Recovery volunteer, upon the request of the physician, visits the patient in the hospital. Many women report that this is extremely helpful, particularly because they feel that by meeting with an active woman who has been in their situation but now looks and feels well, they are encouraged to believe they, too, will make a good recovery.

The volunteer tells the patient about a breast prosthesis (a form that fits into the brassiere), and even brings a temporary one with her. She also demonstrates some of the exercises that help the postmastectomy patient regain muscle strength and mobility.

Many surgeons routinely have a representative from Reach to Recovery visit all their patients undergoing breast surgery for cancer. If your doctor does not mention this program, feel free to mention it to him and say that you would like to see one of these volunteers.

Postmastectomy Rehabilitation

Some hospitals have a program of rehabilitation exercises that begins while the patient is still in the hospital and may continue after discharge. A number of Y's (both YWCA and YWHA) throughout the country sponsor programs, such as ENCORE, that offer rehabilitation exercises and discussion groups. Your physician, nurse, or social worker at the hospital should be able to tell you about any programs offered in your community.

Exercises will be outlined for you by your physician, a nurse, or a physical therapist. These exercises usually consist of upper- and lower-arm isometrics, or hand-squeezing exercises using putty and a sponge ball. Another exercise consists of "crawling the wall" with the fingers of the affected arm, going higher and higher each day.

You will probably be advised to do as much as you can with the affected arm: You can begin the hand-squeezing exercise yourself, using a sponge ball, rolled-up paper, or cloth. Use the affected arm to brush your hair, to towel yourself dry after showering, and to stir foods. You may be told to use the unaffected arm to "help" the affected one do "heavy" work, such as hanging up coats and lifting.

Breast prosthesis. A breast prosthesis is a breast form that fits into a brassiere; it substitutes cosmetically for the breast that has been surgically removed. Major department stores often have a specialist in the lingerie department who can order one for you; in some communities there are stores that specialize in lingerie and bathing suits for the postmastectomy patient. Your surgeon or the nurse or social worker at the hospital may be able to tell you about them. The American Cancer Society, and Reach to Recovery volunteers also usually maintain lists. The Yellow Pages often lists shops that specialize in various postmastectomy supplies, including breast forms, brassieres, bathing suits, sleepwear, and sportswear. Look under the heading Artificial Breasts.

It is important that a prosthesis fit well. It balances your weight, helping you to avoid back, neck, and shoulder discomfort. It also makes your clothes fit properly, and it offers an important psychological boost. If you look well, you will feel better. You are not being self-indulgent if you spend as much as you can to get the "best" prosthesis possible. In many instances, part or all of the cost will be covered by your insurance. The postmastectomy shops or specialists in lingerie departments of some stores can advise you on completing any insurance forms.

Reconstructive breast surgery. Many women choose to have reconstructive surgery after mastectomy. Their reasons vary. Some say it helps them to "forget" the whole cancer experience or that it makes them feel "whole again." Other, more pragmatic women, say it simply makes clothes fit better and eliminates the need to bother with a prosthesis.

Reconstructive surgery is not for everyone—and nobody should be "talked into it." A woman should do it for herself because she wants it, not to please someone else.

Procedures have been developed to reconstruct breasts that are natural to the eye and touch; even women who had a mastectomy many years ago are choosing to have reconstruction today. Most women who have had a mastectomy can have some type of reconstruction.

Your surgeon should ask you, prior to mastectomy, if you plan to have reconstruction, in order to make certain accommodations for it during surgery. It may be difficult to really "know" beforehand how you will feel, so many women prefer to wait before making a decision.

Some surgeons advocate breast reconstruction by a plastic surgeon at the same time as the mastectomy. However many oncologists believe the optimum time for reconstruction should be one to two years after mastectomy in any woman who has had node involvement at the time of her original operation.

Among the several types of reconstructive procedures available, the appropriate one for you will depend upon the type of mastectomy you had, treatment that followed surgery, your type of skin and muscles, and your breast size.

Surgery may be fairly simple or rather complex. Some surgical procedures are done on an outpatient basis; others require several days or a week-long hospitalization; and some are done in stages over a period of six months to a year. A silicone envelope filled with gel or salt water may be implanted in a pocket created under the chest muscle, but other procedures also require the transplant of skin and/or muscle from other parts of the body. Often reconstruction will involve surgical reduction of the other, normal breast.

Before deciding on surgery, you should know that although the procedure is now performed almost on a routine basis, there is a small risk of complication. Some women have an unfavorable, allergic-type response to the implant; others develop an infection. Transplanted skin or muscle can fail to "take," even though it is from the woman's own body.

In the hands of an experienced plastic surgeon, however, your chances for an uncomplicated and cosmetically successful result are excellent. Most cancer experts believe that reconstruction will not cause a recurrence of the cancer.

The surgeon who operated on you for the cancer, or your medical oncologist, can recommend a plastic surgeon to you. You can also contact the American Society of Plastic and Reconstructive Surgeons; they will give you the names of three board-certified plastic surgeons in your area (see Appendix VI). The American Cancer Society and your local medical society may also be able to suggest plastic surgeons who perform reconstruction. You may wish to speak with a few plastic surgeons before deciding with whom you feel most comfortable. This doctor should be able to:

- tell you how long you must wait after mastectomy. (Most doctors want you to wait until chemotherapy and/or radiation are completed.)
- show you pictures of how the reconstructed breast will look, and describe how the reconstructed breast will feel.
- explain how the reconstructed and the remaining breast can be "matched."

- tell you how long you will have to be in the hospital.
- estimate the length of recovery time.
- discuss costs (usual range: $1,200–5,000 for surgery; hospital costs are extra). Most insurance policies pay for all or part of the procedure.
- refer you to other breast-reconstruction patients upon whom he has operated.

THE EFFECTS OF HEAD-AND-NECK SURGERY

Surgical procedures for head-and-neck cancers may result in visible defects of the face, including the eyes, ears, nose, or mouth. Functional defects may also occur, and removal of part or all of the tongue can affect or even prevent speech. But with rehabilitation, many of these patients learn to communicate well. Complete removal of the larynx will result in the permanent loss of normal speech.

Today, many of these defects can be "corrected," permitting the patient to resume normal activities and to have an acceptable appearance. Maxillofacial prosthetics (artificial replacements for missing parts of the face) are remarkably effective. Ears, eyes, parts of a nose or even a complete one, mouth, lips, teeth, and parts of the palate can all be replaced permanently. This type of restorative, reconstructive surgery is usually done in large medical centers; it is planned before the cancer surgery. The surgeon who is going to remove the cancer can discuss the relevant kind of reconstruction with you.

When the larynx is totally removed, an opening is created in the lower front part of the neck. Because there is no longer a connection from the lungs to the mouth or nose, breathing, coughing, and sneezing take place at the new opening. The laryngectomee (as such a patient is called) eats and drinks as usual, but he loses a great degree of the senses of smell and taste, and he no longer can speak as he did.

However, with rehabilitation, the laryngectomee does learn to speak, usually in one of three basic ways. *Esophageal speech* is achieved by taking some air into the mouth and swallowing or forcing it into the esophagus by locking the tongue to the roof of the mouth. When the air is forced back, it causes the walls of the esophagus and pharynx to vibrate, which then allows for a low-pitched sound to be articulated into words as with normal speech. *Pharyngeal speech* is attained by using the small amount of air that goes into the nose and mouth when you breath through the tube in the trachea. This creates a very hoarse, but clearly intelligible speech. Another way is to use a battery-operated device that is held against the neck. Sound travels from this electrolarynx, as it is called, through the neck and into the mouth, where the laryngectomee forms words as usual. The speech has a somewhat mechanical, "robotlike" sound, but is easy to understand.

Prior to surgery, your doctor will discuss the extent of the planned surgery, and will arrange for you to meet with a speech pathologist, who will help you achieve the maximum articulation possible. The American Cancer Society also sponsors organizations such as The Lost Cord and the International Association of Laryngectomees, which help patients and their families cope with the loss of the larynx. (See Appendix VI.)

OSTOMIES

More than a million people in the United States and Canada have had part or all of their colon or bladder surgically removed. Normal functioning thereafter requires an ostomy, the surgical construction of an artificial opening called a stoma. These people continue to lead normal lives, and nobody knows they have an ostomy unless they choose to tell others.

The adjustment to living without a normal rectum or bladder opening is less complicated than many people think, and does not cause you to bulge, smell, make noises, or become a captive of the toilet. Nor does it prevent you from traveling, having sex, bathing, showering, swimming, or participating in most sports.

Urostomies. If the entire bladder is removed by surgery—in a procedure called a cystectomy—a substitute for the storage of urine must be provided. The urinary diversion, called a *urostomy*, is performed by disconnecting the ureters from the bladder and joining them to the end of a small segment of the ileum (part of the small intestine). This segment is converted into a conduit and brought through the wall of the abdomen near the navel, where it forms an opening called a stoma. This enables urine to flow out of the body. An appliance, sometimes called a bag or pouch, is placed over the stoma to collect urine. At night this is connected to a bedside drainage bag with a greater capacity. Recently, some surgeons are creating "internal bladders," which do not require an external appliance. They are emptied with a catheter; the patient learns to do this independently.

Colostomies. A *colostomy* is a surgical procedure performed when parts of the colon and the rectum are removed. A portion of the colon is brought through an opening in the abdominal wall to form the stoma. Fecal matter drains into a plastic pouch. In those instances where the end of the colon is not diseased, the rectum is not removed and the colostomy is temporary; it can be reversed. Colostomies are named after the section of the colon that is operated on. Thus, there are sigmoid (or descending) colostomies, in which the bowel movements resemble those you had before surgery. The discharge from transverse (or ascending) colostomies is semiliquid. Some people with sigmoid colostomies regulate and predict drainage by means of irrigation and diet, so they do not always have to use a pouch.

Ileostomies. An *ileostomy* is performed when the entire colon is removed. The ileum is brought out into the abdominal wall to form the stoma. It may be temporary, but if the rectum is also removed, it will be permanent. An ileostomy causes frequent discharges, so the appliance must be emptied four to six times a day and must be worn at all times. The drainage is semiliquid to liquid. Many patients have "continent" ileostomies. Instead of wearing an external appliance, the patient empties the fecal content through a tube.

Care of Ostomies

Although you can eat the same foods you ate before surgery, some people find that certain foods may cause odors when the appliance is emptied. Foods that cause gas—such as baked beans, onions, cabbage, and asparagus—may be problematic, so you may wish to avoid them. Drinking cranberry juice can be especially helpful in preventing odors from urostomies, because it keeps urine in an acid state. If you have a colostomy, putting an aspirin in the pouch (not the stoma) can help get rid of any disagreeable odors. If you have an ileostomy, chew your food well and avoid peanuts and corn.

Adjusting to the differences in bodily functions caused by an ostomy is not as difficult as you might imagine. Following surgery, nurses will help you with these new functions, but before you are discharged you will learn to do it yourself. In many hospitals a nurse who is an enterostomal therapist (known as an ET) will teach you how to care for it; in some hospitals, other nurses will do this.

Many patients continue to have a visiting nurse come to their home to offer assistance and support until they have completely mastered the technique. Sometimes a family member also learns to help do this. It seems complicated at first, but most people eventually find that their daily care takes only about ten minutes.

Technology improves steadily, and it is possible for everyone to have an appliance that fits well. Today's disposable and reusable appliances make it possible to lead a normal life. The stoma will not show, skin irritations can be kept to a minimum, and odors need not be a problem. You will probably be given some samples of appliances to take home, and the nurse will recommend the best types for your particular ostomy.

An ostomy does not prevent you from a close relationship with your sexual partner and it is not a barrier to sexual intercourse. However, when the rectum is removed, various nerves in some men can be affected and lead to impotence (inability to have an erection). This risk should be discussed with your surgeon prior to surgery.

Generally, you will be able to work, travel, dance, ski, bowl, play golf or tennis, and even swim despite the ostomy. You will be able to wear most of your same clothes (including bathing suits), although extratight clothes and brief bathing suits may create a problem. You can wear seat belts in cars and airplanes, adjusting them to avoid pressure on the stoma.

Ostomy Support

You are not alone with your ostomy—although it may seem that way to you sometimes. There are several kinds of support available to you. In addition to hospital nurses and visiting nurses, there are hundreds of ostomy associations throughout the United States and Canada that are part of the United Ostomy Association. This association acts as a clearinghouse for ostomy information and resources, devoting much effort to education of patients and health professionals. It provides literature, lecture material, audiovisual aids, and new information. See Appendix VI for further information on contacting the association. Your physician, nurse, or social worker—as well as your local ostomy association, American Cancer Society, and the National Cancer Institute—may also be able to give you information on joining a group and getting information. They may also be able to recommend good local ostomy suppliers, and can even recommend an ET (enterostomal therapist) in your area. In the Yellow Pages, under the heading Surgical Appliances and Supplies, you will also find dealers that carry various brands of supplies. Many medical-insurance policies will partially reimburse you for these supplies.

Amputation of a Leg

Some cancers, especially those of the bone, may require the amputation of a leg. Mobility is achieved fairly quickly today, because of the tremendous strides in technology. Often the patient is fitted at the time of the amputation, right on the operating table, with a plaster cast attached to a metal tube and a molded rubber foot. The cast helps keep down the swelling and allows you to get used to a prosthesis. As you begin to heal, new casts are fitted. The permanent leg will probably be hollow and plastic, covered with foam rubber. It will be held on by suction, and its joints can actually duplicate the action of natural joints.

. Amputation is a traumatic operation. Although you may be assured that your rehabilitation will be complete, any loss of a body part is a threat to one's self-image, compounded by the realization that a life-threatening illness has made it necessary.

It may be comforting to realize that thousands of amputees—people who've had cancer or other diseases, or who've been in accidents—have gone on to lead normal lives. They work, exercise (even ski!), marry, have children, and function well. Some choose to use a prosthesis all the time; others just some of the time—and still others choose not to use one at all.

The Effects of Prostate Cancer Surgery

In the section on cancer of the prostate, I discussed the various procedures and said that there is sometimes a risk that impotence may follow treatment. At one time many of the surgical procedures resulted in impotence, but recent advances in techniques have greatly minimized the risk. The testicles are sometimes removed from men who have metastatic prostate cancer, and this will usually cause impotence. For this reason, some men refuse surgery. It is, of course, a decision that a man is free to make, but you will want to know that most men feel they would rather opt for the treatment that offers them the best chance at survival even if it limits their sexual ability.

Many men, with or without a sexual partner, seek counseling at this time. Your urologist may be able to recommend a social worker, psychologist, or psychiatrist who specializes in sexual counseling. Relationships can remain warm, sensuous, and mutually satisfying to a man and his partner. It is even possible to achieve orgasm without an erection. In some instances, it may be possible to have a penile prosthesis inserted that allows a man to have an erection that he would otherwise be unable to achieve.

The Effects of Gynecological Cancer Surgery

Surgery for many gynecological cancers involves the removal of the ovaries and/or uterus, causing a woman to be unable to conceive or bear children. She will go through a surgically caused menopause and change of life; her menstrual periods cease and she may develop symptoms of natural menopause, such as hot flashes.

Some of the surgical procedures for female genital cancers make intercourse uncomfortable or even painful for some time following surgery. Lubricant creams may help, but if there is a shortening or narrowing of the vagina, the physician may recommend you use dilators to stretch it out again.

The complex emotional impact of gynecological cancer is twofold. Cancer itself represents a loss of health; gynecological cancer may represent a perceived loss of femininity as well as some real loss of sexual and reproductive abilities. Such feelings of deprivation may strike a woman even if her appearance has not changed, even if she does not plan to have children in the future, and even if she does not want a sexual partner. Her self-image, both conscious and unconscious, is what matters most.

Recovery from any surgery can take time—and often, changes occur in appearance and functioning that make a person wonder if it's "worth it." But human beings are remarkably adaptable, and most people eventually learn to accept and live with change. In Chapter 16 I will discuss the emotional aspects of coping with cancer and treatment.

Chapter 11
Minimizing and Coping with the Side Effects of Radiation

At one time the side effects from radiation were often severe, but today's machines permit stronger, far more direct doses, which eliminate many of these problems. But still, side effects do exist, and although most of them are confined to the area being treated, some effects can occur throughout the body. Most of them are temporary, usually occurring soon after treatment begins and continuing for a few weeks after completion.

Fatigue is the most common side effect of radiation. Although no one is certain of the reason, some believe it is probably due to the breakdown of tumor cells, their absorption into the bloodstream, and the energy being expended to rebuild injured cells. Although many people continue to work while they are receiving radiation, others find they are very tired and require a great deal of rest. Try not to get discouraged; in all likelihood, you will regain your usual energy level soon after treatment is concluded. Schedule rest periods throughout your day.

Loss of appetite may also occur, followed by weight loss. You may also feel nauseous, if you are getting treatment to the abdomen. (Hints for good nutrition during treatment are given in Chapter 14.) Even if your appetite is poor, try to eat. Here are some suggestions to help:

- Eat whenever you are feeling hungry—even if it is not your usual mealtime.
- Have nutritious high-protein snacks handy to tempt yourself. Fruit, cottage cheese, milk, yogurts, fruit juices, and cereals are easy to fix.

- Try new foods; if you're not in the mood to cook, buy "take-outs" or frozen dinners. Try some new canned soups, and use some of them as sauces over chicken, fish, or toast.
- Eat with someone—family or friends. If that's not possible, consider eating at a counter in a neighborhood eatery where some social exchange takes place. Or take your meals in front of the television, or glance through a magazine or catalog while you are eating.

Skin reactions often occur in the area where treatment has been directed. This is because the radiation must pass through the skin of the treatment area to reach the cancerous cells in the tissues below. Reactions may occur where the radiation enters or leaves the body. Skin will be more sensitive to all irritation, so you should avoid using strong or perfumed soaps, cosmetics, perfumes, colognes, heat lamps, and hot-water bottles. Even with good, careful care, the skin in the treatment area may become red, flaky, itchy, tanned, or sunburned. Applying cornstarch can be soothing.

Hair loss may occur in any area where the radiation is directed. The follicles (pouchlike depressions in the skin from which hair grows) are affected, so although most people identify hair loss with their scalp hair, the beard, mustache, eyebrows, eyelashes, armpits, pubic area, legs, and chest can all be affected if they are in the direct path of the radiation.

Hair usually (but not always) grows back after radiation treatment ends. If a strong dosage has been directed toward malignant cells lying under some hair follicles, they may be completely destroyed. Once follicles are destroyed, there is no regrowth of hair.

Treatment of Specific Areas

Head and neck. Prior to treatment, it is wise to have a dental examination so that any problems can be taken care of before treatment begins. Your dentist may want you to see him regularly during the treatment period so that he can help prevent mild problems from becoming severe ones. He may suggest that you rinse your mouth regularly with salt water (one teaspoon salt and one teaspoon baking soda to one quart of water) or peroxide (one part peroxide to two parts water). He may also recommend flouride applications on a daily basis, and the use of a toothbrush with soft, rounded bristles or even just cotton swabs, to keep your mouth clean and comfortable in this period of heightened sensitivity. (And use toothpaste with flouride and plaque control.)

You may also suffer from loss of taste, and you may develop dryness or small sores in the mouth, difficulty in swallowing, or a lump in your throat. Aspergum or throat lozenges, or glycerine swabs, can be of help. A diet of soft, bland, and well-cooked foods will be easiest to eat at this time. (In Chapter 14 I will discuss the various foods that are easiest to eat and digest during cancer treatment.)

Radiation to the area around the salivary glands may slow down the production of saliva, causing the mouth to be very dry. It is helpful to drink plenty of water and other liquids, rinse your mouth often, suck on ice cubes, and apply wet gauzes. A mouthwash as described above will also help alleviate dryness. (Refrain from using commercial mouthwashes that contain alcohol, because they will only worsen dehydration.) Since reduction of saliva can lead to tooth decay, be sure you check in with your dentist often.

Head. Side effects and pain are usually minimal. Hair loss is usually temporary but *can* be permanent. Steroids are usually given to prevent brain swelling.

Abdomen. Radiation to the stomach, abdominal or rectal area can cause nausea, cramps, urinary frequency, vomiting, and diarrhea. Don't be a martyr—tell the doctor or nurse treating you; they *can* give you medication to control it. You can help to control nausea by eating lightly before and after treatments. (See Chapter 14 for specific hints on diet for nausea and diarrhea.)

Chest. Some people begin to cough after treatment, and jump to the conclusion that they are getting worse. Don't panic—this is, in all likelihood, a side effect from the radiation. If the esophagus is in the field of treatment, you may have difficulty in swallowing or feel as if there's a lump in your throat. A humidifier in your room may be helpful. Also, the doctor can order medications to help the problem and the nurse may have other suggestions.

Pelvis. Cramps, diarrhea, and urinary irritation can occur with radiation to this area. Refrain from hot, spicy foods and follow the other hints given in Chapter 14.

Breast. Side effects from radiation to the breast are somewhat general: Skin reactions and fatigue are the most common. Swelling of the arm (lymphedema) can be caused by radiation to the lymph nodes and vessels. See pages 142–143 for a fuller discussion of this side effect.

Radiation implants. Side effects depend on where the implant is placed, but generally they are similar to the effects from external radiation to the same area. Many people continue to be tired for a while after the implant is removed.

Late Effects of Radiation

Radiation tends to affect the small blood vessels, so the blood supply to some organs can decrease in the months following treatment, but this is a fairly infrequent occurrence.

If a man or woman plans to have children after the treatment is completed, he or she should discuss this with the physician prior to radiotherapy. In some instances a man may be advised to bank his sperm before treatment. A woman may be advised when it is safe for her to become pregnant.

Generally, the side effects of radiation are temporary, starting shortly after treatment has begun and lasting only a short time after it is concluded. The symptoms are often exacerbated by the daily trip to the hospital or office for radiation treatments, especially if you have early-morning appointments. A car or bus ride, for instance, can increase feelings of nausea. Discuss any such problems with the doctor or nurse, because they may have specific suggestions to help you.

Chapter 12
Minimizing and Coping with the Side Effects of Chemotherapy

You may have heard that "the cure is as bad as the disease" and other myths about chemotherapy—but they are really not true (at least not anymore). In the last few years tremendous strides have been made in helping patients tolerate the side effects of the drugs. Even those drugs—such as cis-platinum, which patients have described as horrendous—need no longer be feared.

Some people have no side effects from chemotherapy; others have many. Most have just some, and then only at times.

Side effects—or toxic reactions, as they are sometimes called when severe—are caused because the drugs interfere with normal cell growth. As you will remember from the chapter on chemotherapy, these drugs have a systemic effect, working to fight and destroy cancer cells throughout the body. But they are not always selective, and so will affect normal cells as well. Normal cells regenerate, however, so side effects are usually temporary. Those cells that tend to divide and multiply rapidly are most vulnerable to the side effects of chemotherapy. Thus, the gastrointestinal tract, bone marrow, hair follicles, and skin are usually prime targets for these side effects. Muscles, nerves, and certain sexual characteristics may also be affected.

Although the side effects are temporary, when you are experiencing them, they can certainly seem as if they will never cease. As I have said so often, each patient is unique in his particular disease and response to treatment; likewise, each patient is unique in reaction to the drugs. Also, a certain drug may cause symptoms at one time in a patient but cause none at a later time. Some patients may vomit all day from a particular drug, while another patient receiving the drug may experience only a vague sense of nausea or even eat as heartily as before.

157

There is one important point that bears repetition here. You may have heard that unless you are experiencing side effects, the treatment is ineffective. This is not true. If you are being "undertreated," you may not have any side effects, but even with maximum, optimum, and aggressive treatment that is shrinking your tumor, you may be without these effects. Conversely, if you are having strong side effects, there is no assurance that the drug is working effectively. And some drugs used in cancer chemotherapy simply have few or no side effects.

The oncologist has specific ways of measuring how well the drug is working to shrink, reduce, or control your cancer, but the extent of side effects will not usually be one of them. In the use of some drugs, such as Methotrexate, you may be given larger and larger doses until there are *some* side effects; specifically, sores in the mouth. An antidote may then be administered for such drugs.

A good rule of thumb: *There is no relationship between side effects and drug effectiveness.*

Perhaps more than any other treatment, chemotherapy has been referred to as the "big trade-off." It is often hard to believe that you are getting better if you are feeling sick as a result of treatment. Most of those who have been through it and are experiencing increased survival time, control, or cure of their disease will look back and say they would go through it again. And indeed, even those who said, "Never again" just a few years back do go through chemotherapy again if they have a recurrence. Many of these patients also say that the side effects are not nearly as difficult to tolerate as they were before some of the new anti-emetics (drugs that prevent or alleviate nausea and vomiting) were introduced.

Since side effects do vary from drug to drug and from patient to patient, your doctor may not be able to precisely predict how you will react, but he can and should give you a broad outline of the possibilities. He may also be able to give you some specific suggestions for minimizing, reducing, alleviating, and sometimes even preventing some of the side effects. (See Appendix V for an outline of the side effects of most drugs used today.)

Fatigue

Fatigue and lack of energy are common side effects of chemotherapy, as with radiation. Since chemotherapy seems to go "on and on," this can be upsetting. It is sometimes hard to believe you are getting better when you feel so rotten.

Rather than giving up and saying, "I'm too tired for *anything*," many people say they begin to "prioritize" their activities. That is, they decide what is really important and do that, letting other things go undone if they can't find someone else to do them.

Gastrointestinal Side Effects

Nausea, vomiting, and diarrhea are often caused by chemotherapy. The vomiting control center of the brain is also affected by chemotherapy. Although some medicines do not produce these side effects, most do cause some temporary symptoms.

Nausea, that unpleasant sensation which is difficult to describe to someone who has never experienced it, is commonly referred to as "feeling sick to your stomach." It is often accompanied by dizziness, pallor, and sweating. With chemotherapy, it may occur after treatment, or you may feel chronically nauseous.

Vomiting is often accompanied by feelings of weakness, dizziness, and lightheadedness. Your breathing may become irregular.

You may find that limiting your diet to easily digestible foods, and eating smaller amounts of food often, rather than the usual three meals a day, is more comfortable for you. Eat lightly before treatments.

If you are suffering from nausea and/or vomiting, discuss it with your doctor. He may suggest you take your chemotherapy pills at a different time of the day, and he may also be able to recommend some antinausea medication, which you'll take either before or after symptoms begin. If your gastrointestinal symptoms are really intolerable, your doctor may prescribe a sedative strong enough to allow you to sleep for the several hours after treatment, which is when these symptoms are most likely to occur. If you are already vomiting when you call the doctor, he may prescribe an antinausea medication in suppository form, which you take rectally.

When drugs that usually cause nausea and vomiting are given in a clinic or office setting, you will be given Compazine, Trilafon, Torecan, or another antinausea drug to take at home before your treatment appointment. They are effective, but become far more so when used in combination with the newer antinausea drugs, such as Reglan and Ativan. Your doctor will prescribe these drugs according to your individual needs.

In addition, other drugs—such as corticosteroids in high doses, and Haldol, which is usually thought of as a psychiatric drug—are effective antiemetics for some people. Sedatives like Valium and Dalmane may also be useful. Marijuana or THC (the active ingredient in marijuana) and its derivatives have also been used by doctors to fight nausea. Some recent studies, however, have demonstrated that THC may impair the functioning of cells that have a key role in the body's defenses against disease.

Many doctors admit patients to the hospital for two nights when they are having cis-platinum or some of the other "big gun" drugs, as patients call them. Patients are admitted to the hospital the night before treatment and are allowed to "sleep the treatment through," going home the morning after. Some new antinausea medications are especially effective when given intravenously in high doses. If you have been getting treatment as an outpatient, and have come to dread every session, discuss this option with your doctor. Ask him if he can admit you to the hospital for the treatment so that the antinausea drugs can be more effectively administered.

Nonmedical ways to treat nausea. During the period you are experiencing the effects of treatment, it may be helpful to be with someone who can provide a calm, reassuring presence and help you avoid unpleasant smells or sights, and perhaps talk quietly with you about pleasant things. However, some people who are otherwise social and outgoing prefer to be alone during this period.

Some people become nauseous, and some even vomit, *before* they have a treatment. Just the sight of the parking lot at the doctor's office or clinic (even before you smell the alcohol swabs in his office) can induce this response. Don't think you are crazy if this happens to you: Anticipatory nausea and vomiting are very common. It is a conditioned response, and any sight or smell that you associate with chemotherapy can bring back the physical feelings you experience with treatment. This anticipatory anxiety and nausea *can* be treated. Discuss it with your physician.

Many people have found that listening to favorite music with stereo earphones is enormously helpful. Others find that closing their eyes and thinking about a lovely sight—perhaps a mountain stream, the seashore, or a beautiful garden—can be very relaxing. Some people ask a friend with a quiet, soothing voice to record a ten-minute tape describing such a scene, and they play it when they are feeling the effects from a treatment. You can even tape it yourself. In Appendix VI I list some commercial relaxation tapes you can buy or borrow from a library.

Some patients whose nausea is not too intense find that just getting their mind off the treatment is helpful. They go to a movie, meet with friends, or read a good, fast-moving mystery, romance, or science-fiction book. Others have found that counseling which makes use of behavioral modification and self-hypnosis is very helpful (more about that in Chapter 16).

If you simply have no appetite and are losing weight, your doctor may recommend a food supplement. Sometimes vitamins, hormones, and cortisone derivatives help the appetite. Discuss this possibility with your doctor.

Foods that are easy and quick to eat, such as crackers, plain chicken, and milkshakes, may help you get back into the eating habit. Some of the suggestions for making eating time more appealing are found in the section on radiation in Chapter 11. And in Chapter 14 I will discuss further hints on eating.

Diarrhea. If diarrhea becomes a problem, you should adjust your diet to a minimum of roughage and fiber and place emphasis on foods such as cheese, lean meat, fish, and boiled milk. Drink plenty of fluids to replace the fluids and salts you have lost, and discuss the problem with your doctor, especially if it lasts more than a day or two. He may recommend medication. But do not take any medication for this problem without first talking to him. Your physician may also recommend that you eat frequent meals of smaller amounts. Boiled white rice is good; so are applesauce and bananas; but stay away from other raw fruits, vegetables, beans, corn, onions, grains, and nuts. Diarrhea can cause the loss of potassium, which will make you feel weak. Bananas are high in potassium, as are fish, potatoes, and meat. Your doctor may want to recommend potassium supplements if he feels you have a deficiency.

If the diarrhea causes irritation in the anal area, you can use a soothing ointment. Some patients recommend the ointments used for babies' diaper rash.

Constipation. Some drugs cause constipation, and if that occurs, you should try to stay away from cheeses, puddings made with boiled milk, and other foods that can cause constipation. Instead, eat plenty of fruits, vegetables, breads, and nuts—all of which are high in fiber. Fluids are necessary, and prune juice may be especially helpful. Bran can be added to cereals and casseroles. Raisins are good too. Beware of going to extremes, however, or you'll have diarrhea. If necessary, take a daily stool softener, and perhaps use a suppository. Ask your doctor for other suggestions. But again, do not take a laxative or any medication without first talking to him about it.

Be sure to report constipation to your physician, especially if you also have some numbness or tingling in your fingers or toes. Constipation sometimes accompanies this side effect. In such an instance, the doctor may want to change drugs or adjust dosage.

Effects on Mouth, Gums, and Throat

If you develop a bad taste, dryness, or soreness in your mouth, you may find that the sensation can be relieved with special attention to mouth care. Use a bland (no alcohol) mouthwash or make your own from baking soda and water, and use a soft-bristle brush, cotton swabs, or sterile cotton balls. Special glycerine swabs or a prepared cleansing antiseptic intended for people with canker sores or dental irritations can be purchased in most pharmacies. Milk of magnesia applied to the mouth sores with a cotton-tipped swab may also be comforting. Some anesthetic-type lozenges or sprays may also be helpful. If your mouth is very dry, your doctor can prescribe artificial saliva. If your lips become dry and cracked, use creams and ointments that are intended specifically for chapped lips.

Rinses made of well-diluted salt water, glycerine, or baking soda may be helpful. Be sure the mixture is *carefully* diluted and prepared (one teaspoon to one cup water). Try to drink lots of fluids (avoid citrus juices, which may sting or burn), and eat soft foods that are moistened with gravies, sauces, margarine, or butter. Try experimenting with new food seasonings to enhance food flavors (although most people tend to prefere more bland food than usual if they are having trouble with their mouth or throat).

Make good use of your blender or food processor to soften all foods. You may even wish to try prepared baby foods. Today's baby foods are somewhat tasteless (they no longer add salt or sugar), so you may want to add a bit of your own favorite seasoning. At the risk of sounding repetitious, remember that everyone is different. What may help another patient may not work for you.

Discuss any mouth problems with your dentist, since the reduction of saliva flow can lead to tooth decay. If you are going to have any dental work, be sure to tell your dentist that you are currently receiving chemotherapy. If your dentist says that you require any injections, oral surgery, tooth extractions, or root-canal work, talk to your oncologist. He may want to perform blood counts just prior to these procedures.

Effects on Blood and Bone Marrow

The bone marrow, you will remember, is the soft, spongy material found inside the cavities of the bone. It is here that many of the important components of the blood are made. Since bone marrow multiplies very rapidly, it is especially susceptible to chemotherapy. The effects may be experienced and noticed directly by patients, but more often they are subtle, initially detected by the doctor using routine examinations and blood tests. It is for this reason that your doctor asks you to have blood tests so often during treatment, even if everything seems to be all right. Often, he schedules these tests between treatment sessions.

Bone-marrow depression is a term that refers to the body's decreased ability to manufacture platelets, red blood cells, and white blood cells. Each of these cell types has a specific function; if they are affected by chemotherapy, your physician can take certain corrective measures.

White blood cells (wbc) fight against infection. They are active in response to disease, immunity, and medication. A marked decrease in their supply (leukopenia) can lower your resistance against infection. If your white count is lower than your oncologist feels it should be, he may delay or reduce the dose of your next chemotherapy session.

During certain phases after chemotherapy has been administered, your white blood count may drop, returning later to normal. It is wise for patients undergoing treatment to avoid unnecessary contact with people who have infectious conditions that might be transmitted. If you develop a seemingly unimportant injury or illness—say, a boil or cut— you should discuss it immediately with your medical oncologist. And be sure to report any sign of infection; your doctor may wish to give you antibiotics. Call your doctor if you have:

- Temperature over 100° F.
- Chills.
- Headaches.
- A cough or sore throat.
- Shortness of breath.
- Pain or burning during urination.
- "Loose bowels" or diarrhea.
- Boils, redness, swelling, or a serious cut.
- Nasal or eye infections.
- Rectal or lip sores.
- Bleeding or unusual discharge from genital or rectal area or lungs.

To prevent infections:

- Don't pick at or cut nail cuticles.
- Be careful when cutting fingernails and toenails.
- Stay away from sick people.
- Wash hands well before eating.
- Avoid unnecessary crowds indoors.

If your white blood count is low, don't panic. Natural recovery will probably occur in a few days. If the symptoms persist or increase, your physician may arrange for you to have a transfusion of white blood cells.

Red blood cells (rbc) transport oxygen to tissues, and waste products (carbon dioxide) from tissues. A reduction in red blood cells (low hematocrit) can leave you feeling tired, dizzy, or irritable; or you may experience chills, headache, shortness of breath, as well as an unhealthy-looking pallor. Reduction in red blood cells can cause anemia; in some instances your doctor may recommend a transfusion. Generally, vitamins, taken with iron and other mineral supplements, will be sufficient to keep your count at a satisfactory level.

Blood platelets aid in clotting, and a reduction (thrombocytopenia) can make you more susceptible to bruising, rashes, or bleeding from internal organs, particularly the stomach and kidneys. If your platelet count is low:

- Be careful with tools, razors, kitchen cutlery, and gardening tools. Shave with an electric razor, and wear protective gloves when using tools.
- If you cut yourself, apply pressure to the cut with a clean cloth, paper towel, or hand. If bleeding continues or swelling occurs, call your doctor.
- Avoid burns (use good pot holders or mitts) when cooking.
- To avoid injuring your mouth, clean teeth with a soft-bristle toothbrush or, better yet, cotton swabs.
- Avoid aspirin and aspirin-containing medications, which can interfere with blood coagulation.
- Check with your doctor before drinking alcohol or taking any medication.

Obvious blood in the urine or stool and unusual bleeding from the nose or gums should be reported promptly to your doctor. Unusually dark stools may indicate bleeding and should also be reported. So should an excess of black-and-blue marks. It is important to be aware of potential bleeding symptoms, since they may occur between your regular blood tests.

Despite the problems that may arise from these lowered counts, your physician has many ways of treating you. Rarely, but sometimes if all three counts drop (pancytopenia), you may have to be isolated from all possible germs, and receive a transfusion of red blood cells, white blood cells, and/or platelets.

Don't make the mistake of thinking that these symptoms are a result of the disease rather than a correctable side effect of the drugs. And remember that most of these effects are reversible. Your doctor, after checking your complete blood count, may make a number of suggestions to rectify side effects. Most people are not seriously troubled with them for any length of time.

Hair Loss

When people are told they need chemotherapy, often their first question is "Will I lose my hair?" Hair loss is one of the most dreaded side effects, perhaps because it is so visible and seems to announce to the world, "I am getting treatment for cancer."

Why do so many of the drugs cause hair loss? Because the cells in the hair follicles are among the most rapidly dividing cells in the body, and thus are particularly vulnerable to the interference of chemotherapy. However, chemotherapy does not destroy the follicles, so the hair loss, known as *alopecia*, is only temporary. Regrowth sometimes even occurs before you complete your chemotherapy.

Some drugs cause no hair loss at all, while others may produce mild or unpredictable degrees of hair loss; yet others are definitely expected to cause a marked amount. As with so many other things, there are individual differences in reaction even from the same drugs. In general, though, hair loss usually follows treatment by two to three weeks.

People normally shed up to one hundred (of their approximately one hundred thousand) hairs each day; those hairs are constantly replaced. In patients receiving chemotherapy, hair may fall out at a far greater rate, or it may fail to grow back. Or it may suddenly fall out, sometimes in great clumps over a period of a few days.

Although people usually think of hair loss purely in terms of scalp hair, the hair follicles of the beard, mustache, eyebrows, eyelashes, armpits, pubic area, legs, and chest can all be affected by chemotherapy. Middle-aged men, who expect they will simply join their friends in looking a little bald, are often shocked to realize that under treatment, the sideburns and fringe hair *also* fall out.

Your scalp may become irritated or flaky, and you may find it helpful to use a milder shampoo, and to rub olive oil or baby oil into the scalp.

Psychologically, hair holds a variety of important meanings to people. Men often equate hair with manliness. The loss of scalp, beard, and chest hair can make them feel asexual as well as older and less attractive. Women find the loss of hair a threat to their self-esteem and femininity.

These are very normal and appropriate reactions. Family and friends may tell you, "This is nonsense—your hair will grow back, and in the meantime, you can get a wig." But finding clumps of hair on your pillow in the morning, or on your brush at night, and seeing yourself in the mirror with less than the usual amount of hair, can be traumatic. At a time when you may be worried and anxious about your general health, this hair loss is just "one more assault" against your body. At a time when you may not *feel* like yourself, you don't even *look* like yourself. However, no one has to look bald or balding if they don't want to.

Hair replacement. Women can look very well in inexpensive, ready-made synthetic wigs, which they can purchase in a local beauty parlor, wig store, or department store. Custom-made wigs of natural hair are expensive, and not really necessary, but if a woman wants one, she can get it through her beauty parlor or from a wig specialist. Look in the Yellow Pages, under Hair Replacement, for specialists in wigs for chemotherapy patients. Some women prefer turbans; you can get them in a variety of colors to go with your wardrobe.

Men's synthetic ready-made wigs can look satisfactory but are not as natural-looking as those made by custom designers. A hairpiece (or toupee) will usually look unnatural; it won't blend into sideburns or fringe hair since a man usually loses that, too. Many men wear a baseball or golf hat, or some other kind of hat—if only to protect themselves from the sun or the cold.

Your physician or nurse, a social worker, or local chapter of the American Cancer Society may be able to advise you where you can get a wig at little or no cost, if you cannot afford to purchase one. Attractive women's synthetic wigs start at under fifty dollars; custom-made (natural-hair) ones run a few thousand dollars. Men's wigs tend to be more expensive; the less costly ones look unnatural.

Medical insurance will often pay some compensation toward a wig for people undergoing treatment; in any case, the cost is a medical tax deduction. Your physician can write a note like this:

> This patient is under my care for [type] cancer and consequently is receiving chemotherapy. As a result of chemotherapy, the patient suffers from alopecia. Therefore, it is medically as well as psychologically necessary that [your name] use a prosthesis (wig).

Preventing hair loss. Hair loss from certain drugs can sometimes be minimized slightly or even prevented by using a scalp tourniquet during the intravenous injection of chemotherapy. This tourniquet may prevent the hair follicles from receiving high concentrations of fast-acting drugs. The tourniquet (a small blood-pressure cuff or cloth band) is tied on the head before the injection begins, and left on for about fifteen minutes after the dose is completed. Some patients report using a scalp-cooling technique, making use of ice-packed caps during treatment. These methods do not succeed for all people, or with all drugs, or when a combination of drugs is given in sequence by injection, or when the drugs are taken by mouth.

A number of physicians are opposed to any method that blocks the drugs from going to the scalp, because the scalp (and even the brain) can become a sanctuary for cancer cells. Others feel the method is safe but ineffective, often causing hair loss to occur in patches, which looks even worse than general hair loss.

Most patients say that eventually they decide that hair loss is a reasonable trade-off, and either decide on hair replacement, wear a head covering, or just "go natural." And, of course, it *will* grow back, frequently stronger, more vigorous and of more youthful color and texture than before.

Skin Changes

Skin cells also multiply quickly, so they are often affected by chemotherapy. Sweat glands may be affected and thrown off balance, drying the skin. Some drugs cause localized or generalized rashes, itching, tender fingertips, or dry flaky skin. Dark circles may appear on fingernails; there may be a discoloration where veins show, particularly in the area near where the injections are given.

Your doctor can prescribe medication to apply to your skin, or he can give you pills that will help alleviate the condition. Skin changes, like other side effects, can be minimized or reduced and will usually disappear when treatment is stopped.

Cornstarch and mild skin lotions may be helpful, and dandruff shampoo may also help. Your doctor should be informed promptly of any *sudden* apparent skin changes, no matter how minor they appear.

Effects on Muscles and Nerves

Some drugs can cause muscle weakness and unsteadiness in walking. Sometimes a mild fever (a general side effect) accounts for such temporary, general weakness. Hearing loss, or a ringing in the ears, can also occur. Certain drugs cause tingling or numbing sensation in hands or feet.

Any of these symptoms can be very frightening; a patient may mistakenly conclude that the cancer has spread to the brain or nervous system. Don't assume these symptoms mean that you are getting sicker—but don't assume, either, that they are side effects. Report any symptoms to your doctor, who can determine if they are related to a low red blood count or are simply another side effect of the drug. If he discovers the latter, your physician will assure you that these symptoms will stop when the drug is discontinued or the dosage decreased. Most patients who experience such symptoms are only mildly affected, and some don't even notice them.

Effects on Secondary Sexual Characteristics

Male or female hormones, adrenal steroid derivatives (such as cortisone), and some chemotherapy drugs may cause certain effects on what are called the secondary sexual characteristics.

Women. During chemotherapy, women who were still having regular menstrual periods may find that their cycle becomes irregular, or even ceases. However, it is still possible for you to become pregnant, so do discuss birth control with your doctor. The Pill may interfere with treatment, but barrier methods (e.g., diaphragm, IUD) will probably be acceptable. A woman should not become pregnant while receiving chemotherapy, because the drugs could have a harmful effect on the growth of a fetus. If you want to have a child after chemotherapy is completed, your physician can advise when this is safe for both you and the child.

Women who are premenopausal or menopausal may experience hot flashes or some bleeding while undergoing chemotherapy.

If a woman is receiving male hormones (androgens) and corticosteroids, she may experience some masculinizing effects, such as a slight deepening of the voice and some extra hair growth on her face or body. She may also feel an increase in appetite, sexual desire, and/or muscle strength, and perhaps notice a minor change in body shape. These symptoms usually subside with dose adjustment. The voice change is hardly noticeable; friends may think it is due to a cold or laryngitis. Stay in good shape and treat yourself to a few new outfits—even if they are in the next size!

Many women use depilatories, and some arrange to have their faces waxed at their local beauty salon. Facial-hair removal could probably be considered a legitimate medical tax deduction, and might even be reimbursable by medical insurance. Ask your doctor for a letter similar to the one on page 166.

Some women feel that these changes—especially if they are accompanied by hair loss, and aggravated by the threat of cancer—are a major assault to their self-image. If you are married or have a regular partner, assurances that you are still the person you always were may help to minimize these feelings. It is quite natural to feel temporarily insecure. With time, you will begin to assume the same attitudes you held about yourself, your sexuality, and your relationships to others, prior to cancer and treatment.

If you do not have a regular partner, you may feel hesitant to begin new relationships. Your interest in sex may be increased or decreased, and this may also affect your feelings about yourself. Many women say that in time they relax and resume their characteristic ways of sexually interacting with other people.

Men. Men who are taking female hormones (estrogens) may feel some reduced sexual desire and experience difficulty in achieving erection. Even in small doses, female hormones can cause some enlargement of the breasts (gynecomastia). To avoid this condition, doctors can treat a man's breasts with a small dose of radiation before hormonal treatment begins. The estrogens also cause some lessening of beard and alteration of body shape. Men who are very thin and athletic-looking may tend to gain weight. Some men also feel thinner-skinned. Generally, these changes are hardly noticeable to anyone but the patient himself, and can be minimized if he stays in good shape through diet and exercise.

These slightly feminizing effects occur because the female hormones atrophy (shrink) the testes and reduce the androgens in the body. A man will not, however, develop a high soprano voice, nor will his personality or sexual orientation change. Since he has had a full quota of male hormones throughout his life, and has perceived himself, and been perceived by others, in a particular way, he will find the results of the small dose of female hormones negligible.

Men who have always taken great pride in their ability to financially provide for themselves, families, or friends, and to be physically and emotionally strong, may become upset because their self-image is threatened. These feelings can affect a man's relationship to his wife or any regular partner, as well as to friends, other family members, and even acquaintances.

If a man perceives himself as "less of a person" for any one of a number of reasons, this can also make him question his ability to have sexual relations. Although chemotherapy can reduce a man's sperm count (fertility), most drugs will not affect his ability to have an erection (potency), but worrying about it *can* result in sexual problems.

If you are troubled with these side effects, you should know that they are not unusual, and with time and an understanding partner, they are usually resolved. Discuss them with your doctor, who may then refer you for counseling. Or seek counseling yourself. (See Chapter 16 for more information about this issue.)

Although chemotherapy can reduce fertility, it is still possible for a man on chemotherapy to make a woman pregnant. Therefore, because some drugs may have an adverse effect on sperm (and thus on a potential fetus), you or your partner should use contraceptives. Your doctor is likely to advise you to wait until a year after chemotherapy is completed before planning to become a father.

Sometimes a man's fertility may be *permanently* affected by chemotherapy. If you hope someday to have a family, you should discuss this question with your doctor prior to beginning treatment. It is now possible to freeze sperm before treatment, and then to arrange insemination at any time during or after chemotherapy is completed. Your physician, or a nurse or social worker at the hospital, may have information on sperm banks in your area.

It is reassuring to note that many men and women have conceived healthy children after treatment has been completed.

Pain at Injection Sites

Most people do not experience pain when injected with treatment drugs, although there may be minor stinging pain. The doctor or nurse will advise you to tell them if you experience severe pain or swelling while drugs are infusing. If you feel pain at the site of the injection, and it is followed in a few hours by redness, swelling, or a lump, you should report this immediately to your physician. He may advise you to apply an ice-pack or an ointment, or he may want to see you. Certain medications are more likely to irritate the veins than others.

If you have continual painful irritation in the area around the veins from the repeated injections of chemotherapy, or from blood tests, your doctor may suggest that you have a right-atrial catheter inserted directly into the circulatory system to provide a pathway for medications and for obtaining blood samples. See pages 64–65 for a full description of it. If your doctor doesn't suggest it, speak to him about the possibility.

Other Side Effects

Some people are bothered by fluid retention, resulting in swelling of ankles or puffiness of the face. Steroids are most likely to cause this effect. Your doctor can presscribe a diuretic, which will help to rid the body of excess water. He may also advise you to reduce your intake of salt.

Some chemotherapy, particularly if it includes steroids or hormones, can cause insomnia, increased appetite, weight gain, and/or mood changes (ranging from an almost unrealistic sense of euphoria to a deep depression). Your physician may either adjust the drug or offer suggestions to counteract these effects.

In the case of an acute depression, your family physician or oncologist should refer you to a psychiatrist, who may prescribe (in consultation with your oncologist) medication for this depression. Follow-up counseling with the psychiatrist—or a psychologist, social worker, psychiatric nurse, or other counselor trained in working with cancer patients—will help you get back to being your "old self."

Some drugs can cause bladder irritation or kidney problems. Your doctor will instruct you to watch for these signs and be prepared to treat them if they develop. You can usually eliminate this problem by increasing your intake of fluids. One drug, adriamycin, can also cause heart problems. Again, you will be carefully monitored, with frequent electrocardiograms, if your doctor is concerned.

Some drugs can change the color or odor of urine. For instance, adriamycin can turn urine red, and methotrexate can turn it a deep bright yellow. There is nothing to worry about, but do call such changes to the attention of your doctor or a nurse.

People say they frequently, or even consistently, feel as if they have the flu; they experience a generalized achiness and sometimes mild fever and chills.

Any symptom or complaint that lasts more than a few days may be a side effect of a drug that you are taking, and should be reported to your doctor. *Don't* assume that you have a recurrence of the disease or that the symptom is another medical problem. Call your doctor anytime you have a fever of over 100°F, rashes, chills, persistent or intense pain (including headaches), shortness of breath or difficulty in "catching" your breath. All these symptoms are reversible and should be investigated. Also see Appendix II, "When to Call Your Physician."

Side effects of chemotherapy are troubling, and no one should make light of them. And they may continue during the entire period of chemotherapy, which can cover a period of several years. Patients sometimes say that their doctors and nurses keep emphasizing the trade-off as if they were unaware of how chemotherapy interferes with and intrudes upon their lives. These patients describe how terrible even the anticipation of treatment can be.

The side effects are often tolerable, but many times they are not. And sometimes they are not fully reversible. As one patient said, "It's a rotten deal, but what choice do I have?"

For many people, however, it's not too rotten a deal. They continue to work, play tennis and golf, bowl, drive a car, and follow their usual pursuits with only slight adaptations in their life-style. And they survive the treatment, and the cancer. You may well be one of these people.

Chapter 13
Pain Management

More than anything else, pain is the most feared aspect of cancer, although most cancer patients do not experience any significant pain. Today much is known about how to interfere with the pain-perception center in the brain, making it possible to effectively control pain.

Although pain can be relieved, many people, including health professionals, family, and patients themselves, often hesitate to take the necessary measures to do so. Fear of drug addiction is often cited (more about that later).

This reticence to deal with pain may hark back to the ancient belief that pain was a result of offending the gods. In more recent years, it has been seen as a "deserved punishment"; patients often say, "What did I do to deserve this?" We tend to admire stoic patients who are able to "take it," as if it is a virtue to endure pain. Such widespread attitudes and social conditioning often restrain the physician from prescribing adequate pain medication, make pharmacists hesitate to dispense the prescription in its entirety, and sometimes keeps nurses and family from giving enough of it. And even when the medication is offered, the patient often refuses to take it. But pain *can*—and should—be managed.

Everyone knows what pain is. It is a sensation that hurts enough to make you uncomfortable. But it is also a message from your body to the nervous system—sort of an alarm that says, "Something is wrong." Pain occurs when damaged or hurt tissue starts the alarm signal, in the form of an electrical impulse through the spinal cord to the thalamus, the sensory center in the brain. From there it goes to the cortex, the brain's outer layer. At that point a person is able to perceive the intensity and location of the pain. Pain is diminished when the brain sends signals down through the spinal cord, releasing such chemicals as endorphins (the body's own morphine), which diminish the pain.

Essentially, there are three types of pain: acute, chronic, and phantom-limb.

Acute pain is experienced as an "event," and may be brief and mild, or severe and extended. Acute pain can be protective, serving to warn us to take measures to remove the cause of it. This kind of pain is associated with surgery or a sudden injury and is usually relieved by analgesics (pain relievers).

Chronic pain can be mild or severe; it lasts a long time, serving no useful purpose. Chronic pain is all-consuming, difficult to tolerate, and can lead to anxiety, depression, loss of appetite, exhaustion, sleep disturbances, irritability, reduced sexual desire, withdrawal from social interaction, unrelenting anger, and preoccupation with the body to the exclusion of all else. These effects, in turn, can worsen the pain, complicating treatment.

Phantom-limb pain. If you have had a limb (or a breast) removed, you may feel a sensation that seems to be emenating from the absent limb. This pain can be excruciating, and although it is a perplexing phenomenon, it is thought by some experts to be related to muscle spasms at the site of amputation. Biofeedback (see page 85) has been helpful in treating phantom-limb pain.

Causes of Pain

In cancer patients, pain may be caused by:

- Pressure or irritation on nerve endings by a tumor or inflammation.
- Penetration of tumor cells into nerves and blood vessels.
- Obstruction of hollow areas by tumor or cancer cells.
- Infections.
- Blocked blood vessels, causing poor blood circulation.
- Cancer cells in the bones, causing pressure.
- Bone fractures caused by cancer cells in the bones.
- Stiffness from inactivity.
- Side effects from chemotherapy and radiation, including constipation, mouth sores, nerve damage, skin inflammation, and muscular pain from vomiting or diarrhea.
- Fear, depression, and anger, which lead to stress and tension, causing discomfort to escalate into pain.
- Chemicals released by a tumor that affect the nervous system.

New theories about the origins of pain perception have led to new attitudes about, and ways of treating, pain. The gate-control theory states that only a limited amount of information can be sent along the spinal cord and nervous system to the brain at one time. As soon as the limit is reached, a "gate" closes, and no more information goes through. When pain signals are sent along the same channels of the nervous system to compete with other (nonpain) information, the gate closes before the pain message reaches the brain.

This explains why people who are very involved in what they are doing (such as a rescue effort) may fail to notice when they have injured themselves. It is also one explanation of how rubbing a sore finger or toe or kissing a child's sore knee actually relieves the pain.

It is known that some powerful pain-blocking chemicals, such as endorphins, occur naturally in the brain, and they can "turn off" the pain signals.

Who Treats Pain?

The best method of pain management is to treat the cancer. Cancer that regresses will often result in alleviation of pain, especially if it was caused by pressure from a tumor.

But that may not always be the case. In that event, you might expect your medical oncologist to simply write a prescription for pain, having at his command considerable knowledge about how to relieve severe chronic pain. However, pain management is such a complex science that he may not be totally familiar with everything that is available today, so he could refer you to specialists in pain management. These specialists are located at many major medical institutions, particularly those that treat cancer patients.

The pain-management team typically consists of neurologists, internists, radiotherapists, anesthesiologists, psychologists, laboratory researchers, nurses, pharmacists, social workers, physical therapists, and occupational therapists.

These specialists tailor drugs, dosage, timing, and route of administration, as well as using nonmedical methods to treat pain, such as hypnosis and relaxation. Just as each patient is unique in his response to treatment, so is each patient's body chemistry unique. There are no predetermined optimal doses or combination of drugs and nondrug treatment that work for everyone. You and the pain-management professionals will be able to work together, sometimes on a trial-and-error basis, until pain is controlled. Remember: It *can* be controlled.

In many medical settings, there is no pain-management specialist. In these settings, patients are often undertreated for pain, because doctors may underestimate the dose or frequency that is needed to control pain.

But just as your family doctor or oncologist can consult with cancer specialists anywhere in the country by phone, so, too, can he consult with pain-management experts at nearby cancer hospitals; or he can contact the American Society of Anesthesiologists Committee on Pain Therapy. If you feel that your pain is not being sufficiently controlled, ask him to do this.

The Patient Is the Best Judge of Pain

How does your doctor know you have pain? He doesn't unless you tell him. Nobody can, with any accuracy, say to you, "You *don't* have pain." Pain is whatever you say it is, and it exists whenever you say it does. You are not a coward or weakling because you have pain. Nor are you a hero for putting up with pain, or a complainer because you don't want pain interfering with the quality of your life.

Pain is especially distressing because it can fill you and those who care about you with a sense of helplessness. So tell the doctor or the nurse, or ask your family to tell them, if you have pain. But try to explain your pain so that the doctor can clearly understand and treat it appropriately. Be prepared to tell your physician the following:

- Location of pain.
- When pain began.
- Type of pain: sharp, dull, throbbing, or steady.
- If the pain stays in one place or moves around.
- Frequency of pain: after eating, times of day, constant, or intermittent.
- On a scale of 1 to 10, the severity of the pain.
- Anything you notice that relieves the pain.
- Anything you notice that worsens the pain.
- Medications you have tried for the pain.
- Methods of pain relief you have used in the past.
- Anything that accompanies the pain, such as nausea or dizziness.

Many patients or family members write down some of this information, keeping a sort of diary of the pain. You or your family may notice that there is a specific pattern that can be altered. For instance, if you tend to have pain in the afternoon, this might be a good time to take something that helps you sleep, so that you will be rested in the evening and can enjoy company or television. However, if you find that your pain is relieved by having visitors, you may want to plan to socialize at that time.

Sometimes pain can be minimized with such improvisations, but remember: It is not a sign of weakness to seek professional help in treating discomfort and pain.

The Effects of Pain

Just as emotions can exacerbate pain, so pain can cause many emotionally charged reactions. It is not at all unusual to become depressed, angry, and lethargic when you suffer pain. It is a rare human being who, suffering from pain, becomes more animated, loving, and productive. That seems to happen only to saints and characters in books and movies.

Many people who experience pain will also have associated symptoms. Nausea, headache, dizziness, tiredness, constipation, and diarrhea can all accompany pain. Pain can interfere with sleep and the ability to eat. It can interfere in many ways with your personal life. For these reasons, it is important to relieve the pain.

ANALGESICS: WAYS TO ELIMINATE PAIN

A number of medical methods to eliminate pain can be employed, some separately and others in combination. Nonnarcotic pain relievers, narcotics, antidepressants, tranquilizers, central-nervous-system stimulants, steroids, and alcohol all have a role. In addition, nerve blocks, neurosurgery, biofeedback, diversion, relaxation, hypnosis, and acupuncture all can help relieve pain.

Nonnarcotic Pain Relievers

Many over-the-counter oral analgesics, such as aspirin and acetaminophen (better known as Tylenol or Datril), can effectively relieve mild to moderate pain. Aspirin, in particular, can reduce swelling and inflammation, but it can also cause stomach upsets and interfere with blood clotting. For this reason, patients undergoing chemotherapy are often told to avoid aspirin, as well as various medications that contain aspirin, such as Excedrin. Some prescription drugs, such as Percodan and Empirin with codeine, also contain aspirin, and can have the same effect as aspirin.

Acetaminophen does not usually cause any side effects (although prolonged use can affect the liver or kidneys), but it is not as effective as aspirin in reducing swelling.

Some anti-inflammatory drugs—such as the prescription drug Motrin or its milder nonprescription forms, like Advil or Nuprin—are often used to relieve muscle and other pain in cancer patients.

Although many of the nonnarcotic pain relievers can be purchased without a prescription, you should still check with your doctor before taking them, especially if you are on chemotherapy. See Appendix III for a detailed list of medications that require a go-ahead from your doctor.

There are also a number of other strong prescription drugs, often combined with narcotics. According to many pain experts, most of them are no more effective than analgesics like Tylenol (which is why your doctor might tell you that Tylenol taken on a specific schedule may be sufficient for repressing pain).

Narcotic Pain Relievers

Narcotics are those analgesics that are derived from opium or are synthesized to act like it. Frequent side effects of these pain relievers are drowsiness, nausea, and vomiting. They can also be habit-forming.

Some of those most often prescribed for moderate to severe pain are:

Codeine
Meperidine (Demerol)
Morphine
Oxycodone (Percodan and Percocet)
Heroin
Levorphanol (Levo-Dromoran)
Hydromorphone (Dilaudid)
Oxymorphone (Numorphan)
Methadone (Dolophine)
Pentazocine (Talwin)
Naluphine (Nubain)
Butophanol (Stadol)
Propoxyphene (Darvon)

Some of these drugs are used alone or in combination with other prescription or over-the-counter pain relievers. They may be administered by mouth (pills or liquid), injection, rectal suppository, or intravenously.

Heroin. You may have heard that heroin is widely used in England to relieve severe pain, but is against the law in the United States. According to those who advocate its use, heroin is superior to morphine and other narcotics, working faster and giving greater relief through a smaller dose. Most experts at major teaching hospitals don't agree, arguing that heroin is less effective than certain other synthetic opiates, such as Dilaudid. They say that heroin is essentially no different from morphine, because once it enters the body, it is rapidly converted into morphine.

Side effects. Narcotics relieve pain, but they are not always free of side effects. Drowsiness, constipation, dry mouth, nausea and vomiting are the most common side effects. Tell your doctor or nurse about it; often, changing to another medication will solve the problem. Some of the side effects can also be controlled.

Drowsiness may be the result of other medications, such as tranquilizers, or may be your body's response to pain relief, allowing you to catch up on missed sleep. Once the pain is relieved, your doctor may lower the dose of the narcotic, which will still be effective but no longer cause tiredness. He may also recommend a stimulant, like caffeine-containing beverages, or prescribe a medical stimulant such as Dexedrine or Ritalin.

Constipation can often be helped by diet—see tips in Chapter 14. Or you may, with the advice of your physician, take a laxative. (Do not take either a laxative or a stool softener without asking him.)

A dry mouth is often relieved by drinking water and other liquids, eating moist foods, rinsing often, or sucking on ice chips. Make a mouthwash composed of baking soda and warm water, and avoid commercial alcohol- or salt-based mouthwashes.

Nausea and vomiting are often helped by antiemetics prescribed by your physician. If walking around or even sitting up seems to cause dizziness and nausea, try staying in bed for a while after you take the narcotic. Nonprescription medicines for motion sickness may help, but ask your doctor before you take any.

Fear of addiction. Addiction is the compulsive and usually escalating use of narcotics to meet physical, emotional, and psychological needs. The drug addict develops behavioral changes, a craving for the drug, and personality disorders. This rarely occurs in cancer patients, according to those who specialize in pain management. They say that less than 1 percent of those treated for pain are at risk of becoming an addict.

When cancer patients have their pain adequately relieved through proper management, they do not exhibit the traits of the addict, and their dosage needs do not necessarily increase. The body may develop some tolerance to the drug, requiring more of the narcotic to relieve the pain, but this is not the same thing as addiction. When pain disappears and the cancer patient no longer needs pain relievers, he may experience the symptoms of withdrawal, but he *will* be able to stop taking the drug, if he slowly tapers off the dosage. In this situation, tolerance and physical dependence do *not* mean that drugs are being abused.

It is unfortunate that so many physicians and families hesitate to give cancer patients sufficient medication to relieve pain—and when such help is offered, patients are foolish to refuse it.

Frequency of doses. Anxiety plays an important role in chronic pain, so anything that can reduce anxiety can help to alleviate pain. Patients who receive pain medication on a schedule and *before* pain recurs have less anxiety and often require lower doses.

Conventionally, narcotics are given only when the patient asks for them, but pain-management experts now know that it is easier and far more effective to prevent pain from recurring than to stop it after it has begun. Treatment often begins with a small dose, which is then increased to the level where it is effective. Each succeeding dose is given before the previous one has worn off. This kind of proper dosage and timing offers the patient excellent control for pain.

Some medical centers allow certain patients to participate in a self-medication program. Patients learn to monitor their own needs, administer and keep track of medications. Such programs can help ease the transition from hospital to home, and allow a patient to be in control of his pain rather than submitting to it.

Other Forms of Relief

Tranquilizers can make you feel more relaxed, and more able to cope with pain. By themselves, or in combination with analgesics, they can reduce pain.

Physicians often prescribe *stimulants and antidepressants* along with certain pain relievers to increase the effectiveness of the analgesic and also to prevent drowsiness.

Alcohol—in moderate amounts—can sometimes offer pain relief, increase appetite, reduce anxiety, and help you get to sleep. But when combined with certain drugs, it can lead to serious, even dangerous problems. Before drinking alcohol, be sure to discuss it with your doctor.

Some patients report that *marijuana* has reduced their anxiety and relieved their pain; others say it has increased it. For those in whom marijuana acts to reduce anxiety, it may be helpful. As I said earlier, however, some recent studies indicate that it may contribute to lowering immunity. Although THC (the active ingredient in marijuana) is sometimes legally available to patients, you should consult your doctor before using it in any form.

Implantable pump. Getting just the precise dosage of pain medication at the proper time can be accomplished with a newly developed implantable medication pump, about the size of a hockey puck, which holds medication and delivers it through a catheter to a specific area of the body, such as the spinal cord. These implantable systems usually consist of a hermetically sealed reservoir, a precise pumping mechanism, and a self-contained energy source, all linked together with a soft catheter. The medication can be meted out at a constant or programmed rate; in other instances, it can be administered by the patient himself as needed. The pump can hold a few months' supply of medication; it is refilled by injection through the skin. Adjustments are made externally by radiofrequency waves. Some of these pumps are totally implantable, usually beneath the skin of the abdomen; others are worn next to the body.

Radiation can be effective in treating pain in some types of tumors in certain locations. A small amount of radiation directed at the bones can offer significant relief for many patients, and can reduce a tumor that is pressing on a nerve.

Chemotherapy and hormones. Even when these treatments cannot cure the cancer, they can often shrink tumors, affording much relief from pain and discomfort.

Nerve blocks. A nerve block is a procedure in which a substance, such as alcohol, cortisone, phenol, or an anesthetic, is injected into or around a nerve, blocking the pathway between the nerve and spinal cord. A nerve block may offer temporary or permanent relief. It is performed by an anesthesiologist or neurosurgeon.

Neurosurgery can offer excellent control for severe pain. In one procedure, called a *rhizotomy*, the surgeon cuts a nerve close to the spinal cord. In another, called a *cordotomy*, a bundle of nerve fibers in the spinal cord is destroyed with an electrified needle. Destruction of those nerves that transmit pain eliminates the pain. Because the patient no longer feels pain, pressure, heat, or cold, he may be at risk of burns or injuries, since he will no longer receive a "warning."

Biofeedback techniques help you to recognize, modify, and control certain involuntary habits or bodily responses. Biofeedback can be helpful to cancer patients who are suffering from the anxiety, tension, and muscle pain that may be a reaction to the disease and its treatment, helping them to relax, and minimizing discomfort.

Acupuncture is a technique in which thin needles are inserted into the body at specific pain-relief points, at various depths and angles. It can stimulate the nerves that suppress pain perception and it can also release endorphins, the body's own morphine. Many people find acupuncture extremely helpful for pain associated with many conditions, and it may be helpful for cancer patients—but use it *only* with your oncologist's consent.

Skin stimulation makes use of pressure, heat, cold, vibration, electrical stimulation, or menthol preparations. Generally, the appropriate stimulant is applied to or near the painful area, or in some instances on the opposite side of the body. You should not use any of these methods without first discussing them with your oncologist. If you are presently receiving, or have just completed, radiation treatment, these techniques are *not* for you.

Pressure can be applied in various ways. Massage, using a slow, gentle, circular motion, can relax you, reducing pain. Pressure firmly applied to the painful area, or to a "trigger point" near the pain, can be effective for a considerable period of time. Battery or electric vibrators, held to the head or lower back, can diminish pain there.

Heat, in the form of a conventional or moist-heat electrical heating pad, hot-water bottle, wet towel, hot bath or shower, can ease soreness in muscles.

Cold can offer faster and longer-lasting relief from pain than heat can. Purchase gel packs (from a pharmacy or medical-supply store) that remain soft and pliable when placed in the freezer, or fill a plastic bag with ice cubes. To avoid extremes of cold, wrap the ice packs in a towel before applying to the skin.

Menthol-based creams, lotions, liniments, or gels (such as Ben-Gay) can be gently rubbed into the skin in painful area. Menthol relieves pain by increasing blood circulation.

Electrical stimulation to nerves, in a procedure called *transcutaneous electric nerve stimulation (TENS)*, is a successful method for treating localized pain. The patient wears a small battery-powered pack or box, no larger than a cigarette pack. Electrodes from the box are placed on the skin at various "trigger" points. When you feel pain, you switch on the mild electrical current, for anywhere from five to thirty minutes. It feels like a buzzing, tingling, or tapping. TENS will temporarily block the pain, often giving hours of relief. Patients can wear the device continuously, at or away from home. TENS is usually used in conjunction with other treatments.

If your physician agrees to let you make use of skin stimulation, take the following precautions:

- Avoid extremes of heat or cold.
- Do not go to sleep with a heating pad if you are alone.
- If your circulation is impaired, do not use heat or cold.
- Heat can cause bleeding; do not apply it to an injured area.
- Menthol should not be used on irritated skin, inside the mouth, around the rectum, or near the eyes.
- Do not apply heavy pressure, vibration, or massage over tender or swollen areas.

- Do not continue any skin stimulation if it seems to increase pain.
- Do not use deep and heavy massage in areas where cancer cells may lie, without first discussing it with your oncologist.

Hypnosis puts a patient into a passive, trancelike state resembling normal sleep, during which perception and memory are altered, permitting him to respond to suggestions. Suggestions for the posthypnotic period can also be made during hypnosis. In a less formal fashion, hypnosis also describes a form of arousal or focused concentration during which there is no awareness of what is going on around you, where you are, or what time it is. Many people spontaneously enter an almost hypnotic trance while watching a movie or reading a book.

Because hypnosis allows the mind to ignore involuntary body responses, awareness of pain can be blocked and replaced with a more positive feeling. Many psychotherapists use hypnosis on cancer patients, also teaching them self-hypnosis to control pain. However, this method of pain management has limitations; it does not work for everyone, and it cannot control severe chronic pain.

Your physician can probably refer you to someone who is trained and specializes in hypnosis. Or you can call your nearest pain clinic. See Appendix VI.

Diversion, imagery meditation, and relaxation. Anything that can take your mind off of pain can actually help to relieve the pain. Some people busy themselves with tasks, conversation, a good book, television, or just listening to favorite music.

Others find that imagery and relaxation techniques, including yoga or meditation, help to minimize pain. Relaxation techniques can provide a means of achieving muscle and mind relaxation, shifting attention away from anxiety, pain, and nausea, all of which can interact, exacerbating each sensation.

Pain does not have to be part of living through cancer. Most cancer patients never experience significant pain, and those who do can have it controlled. Be patient; it sometimes takes a little while to find the proper means or the medication, dosage and timing.

Chapter 14

Nutrition: An Ally in the Fight Against Cancer

Nutrition can play an important part in your recovery, along with the rest of your prescribed treatment plan. No special diet, vitamins, or extra attention to nutrition *alone* will cure you or serve as an alternative to proven methods of cancer treatment. A well-balanced diet—one that is high in protein, minerals, and iron—*is* important during treatment, and can help you to fight your cancer. It can also be an enormous help in making you feel better despite the disease.

A recent study shows that cancer patients have a greater chance of making a good recovery from surgery and drug and radiation therapy if their nutrition is improved before and during treatment. In some instances, diet alone cannot achieve these results, and some of the food supplements and other methods I discuss later may be needed.

It is important to note here that some of the fad diets base their treatments on the belief that by depriving a patient of a great deal of nutritional support, they are also halting the growth of the tumor. But cancer experts are firm in their belief that patients receive adequate nutrition, while at the same time receiving appropriate treatments to shrink or destroy the tumor.

It has long been noticed that cancer patients have a tendency to lose weight, and the reasons are still not completely known. One theory is that people who have cancer simply do not feel well, lose their appetite, and eat less. Some studies have shown that cancer also alters metabolism; to feed and enrich the tumor, it robs healthy tissue of needed energy. Thus, the cancer patient's nutritional requirements exceed those of someone without disease. This occurs, unfortunately, just at a time when they feel like eating less than usual, either from the disease or from treatment. As I discussed in Chapters 10 through 12, changes or loss of taste; fatigue; and gastrointestinal effects can all limit your desire to eat.

For these reasons, oncologists often prescribe certain vitamin supplements and advise patients to "eat better" during treatment periods. Because nutrition is not an area in which all oncologists are expert, they often refer patients to nutritionists or registered dietitians for specific recommendations. Your doctor may also suggest that you consult some good diet and menu books for cancer patients. (For a list of some excellent booklets and books on the subject, see Appendix VII.)

Basic guidelines for good nutrition can be adapted for the cancer patient who is experiencing temporary or permanent problems in taste, appetite, digestion, mouth irritation or pain, or who is too tired to eat much at one time. Getting the most nutrition for the least effort is often a sensible goal.

BASIC NUTRITION

Everyone—but especially cancer patients—should try to choose foods from all four of the following groups:

1. Meat, fish, poultry, and other protein foods or substitutes provide protein for building new tissue and replacing cells that may have been weakened by chemotherapy or radiation. Protein is also a good source of iron for blood formation, and for carrying oxygen to help in the production of energy. People who have been ill or had surgery need extra protein for repair, and to help the body defend itself against infection. Patients who are undergoing chemotherapy or radiation are often encouraged to double their normal protein requirements.

These foods contain other minerals and vitamins as well. You should have two servings daily (2 ounces or more per serving) of:

- Meat (beef, pork, lamb, veal).
- Poultry (chicken, turkey, duck).
- Fish (including shellfish).
- Eggs (two medium-size).
- Peanut butter (4 tablespoons, plus a grain product such as bread or crackers) and other nuts.
- Lentils, dried peas, dried beans (1 cup, plus a grain product, such as bread, rice, barley, or crackers; or 1 cup cooked cereal plus cheese or milk).
- Hard cheese (3 ounces or 3 rounded teaspoons).
- Tofu (soybean curd and other soybeans).

2. Enriched/whole-grain breads, cereals, and other grain products provide vitamin B, which aids in appetite and digestion; and carbohydrates and iron, which give energy and help in nutrient absorption and utilization. Also included are other beneficial minerals and vitamins. You should have four or more servings every day of one or more of the following:

- Hot cooked cereals.
- Cold cereals (e.g., wheat, corn, or bran).
- Breads (enriched or whole-grain, such as whole wheat, rye, brown).
- Crackers (e.g., Saltines, graham, melba, pretzels).
- Pancakes, waffles, and crepes.
- Pastas.
- Rice.
- Beans (chick peas; kidney, soy, black beans; lentils; baked beans).

3. Fruits, fruit juices, and vegetables are good sources of vitamin A and vitamin C. Vitamin A helps in the maintenance of mucous membranes (which may be affected by radiation or chemotherapy) and aids in the body's defense against infection. Vitamin C is vital for tissue construction and repair, wound healing, and also as a defense against infection. Fruits and vegetables are also good sources of other vitamins and minerals, and when eaten raw or slightly cooked, they provide fiber.

You should have four servings daily of fruits and/or vegetables. At least one serving should be high in vitamin A and one in vitamin C.

These foods are high in vitamin A:

- Fruits: apricots, cantaloupes, peaches.
- Vegetables: yellow-orange and dark green leafy vegetables, such as carrots, pumpkin, romaine lettuce, spinach, squash, sweet potatoes, broccoli, brussels sprouts, cabbage, celery, cucumbers, green beans, lima beans, okra, green peppers, spinach, turnip greens, tomatoes, yams.

These foods are high in vitamin C:

- Fruits: citrus fruits, such as oranges, grapefruit, lemons, limes; melons, pineapple, strawberries.
- Vegetables: broccoli, green peppers, tomatoes, potatoes.

4. Milk products provide vitamins A, B, and D; protein for energy; and calcium, which builds bones and teeth, helps in blood clotting, and maintains normal muscle tone and nerve relaxation.

You should have two servings daily of milk (1 cup each). It can also be used for cooking: in sauces and soups, on cereals, and in desserts. If milk seems to be causing diarrhea or gas, you may want to try cheese, yogurt, buttermilk, or cooked-milk products instead.

Spreads, sauces, and other fats, though not part of the basic four food groups, have a high energy content to help maintain body weight and give energy. They add flavor to foods. These spreads and sauces lubricate food and are especially helpful if swallowing is difficult. They can be used in cooking and, since they are high in calories, can be helpful if you need to gain weight. Included are:

- Butter, margarine, cooking oil.
- Cream, half-and-half.
- Sour cream.
- Cream cheese.
- Mayonnaise, salad dressings.
- Gravies, dessert toppings.

Minimum Daily Calorie and Protein Requirements

To attain and then maintain your desirable weight, men should multiply that weight by eighteen, and women by sixteen, to determine their minimum daily calorie requirement. If you have been losing weight, men should increase that requirement to twenty times their desirable weight, and women to eighteen times.

Daily protein requirement (in grams) can be determined by multiplying desirable weight by 0.5; if you have been losing weight, multiply by 0.7. (Some nutritionists believe that protein should be increased even more drastically during the period that you are receiving treatment.)

At the end of this chapter is a chart that lists calorie and protein counts of some high-calorie foods you can add to your regular diet in order to gain weight. If you are losing weight, or are low in energy, your doctor may ask you to list all the foods you eat. Use this chart to determine if you are getting sufficient protein and calories.

Tips for Increasing Calorie and Protein Intake

If you need to gain weight, make use of some of these special tips for increasing calories and protein when you really don't want to, or can't, eat more:

- Sprinkle cheese on vegetables, meats; add to casseroles, salads.

- Add skim-milk powder to regular liquid milk, or blend into soups, casseroles, mashed potatoes, puddings, etc.
- Spread butter or margarine on bread; melt into cereals, vegetables, soups, etc.
- Serve ample gravies and sauces over foods.
- Add sugar, honey, syrup, jams, jellies, peanut butter, sour cream, yogurt, cream cheese to cereals, bread, pound or sponge cake, or mix into various soft foods such as custard and yogurt.
- Use a "heavy hand" with the ice cream when making a milkshake.
- Use milk instead of water for reconstituting canned soups.
- Have a granola or candy bar.

LOSS OF APPETITE

It is not at all unusual to lose your appetite during treatment for cancer. It may be the result of illness, fatigue, pain, stress, depression, anxiety, loss of taste, or a combination thereof.

Don't feel you have to force yourself to eat. Try to eat small amounts more frequently or at times when you are feeling your best, even if this isn't your usual mealtime. Flexibility is the key to increasing your nutritional intake. If one week you feel like eating nothing but chicken, then eat as much chicken as you want. Frequent small meals, small portions that do not appear overwhelming, high-calorie snacks, and easy-to-prepare meals will all aid in maintaining sufficient nutrition even when you aren't in the mood to eat. Although they add needed calories, you may find you need to avoid fatty foods such as butter, cream, and salad dressings because they are harder to digest, and can make you feel full.

Keep plenty of convenience foods in the house. When friends or neighbors ask how they can be of help, ask them if they would make up some individual packages of your favorite nutritional foods for you to freeze. Thus, you will be prepared when you do feel hungry.

Sometimes a little mild exercise—or, if your doctor agrees, a glass of wine or beer before mealtime—can increase your appetite.

Change or Loss of Taste

Many people who are receiving chemotherapy or radiation to the head or neck complain that food seems to have "lost its taste." This is due to a common condition called "mouth or taste blindness."

Frequently, for instance, patients say that red meats taste bitter. If this happens, try soaking or cooking it in soy sauce, fruit juice, or wine. Add creamy gravies. Or simply substitute other foods that are high in protein.

Other aversions may develop. Eggs, fish, poultry, or tomatoes may taste bitter, rancid, cottony, or metallic. Substituting plastic cutlery for metal may help. Occasionally, zinc deficiency can alter taste; discuss the possibility of a zinc supplement with your physician.

If such taste aversions do develop, try to eat bland foods with no odors. If you simply find that you have little or no taste, try to arrange food in a pleasing way on the plate. Appetite can be stimulated by appearance as well as taste.

Dry Mouth

Dry mouth is a common side effect of chemotherapy and radiation and is more annoying than it is painful. Your physician may prescribe one of a number of commercially produced artificial salivas. Rinse your mouth as often as you wish—and don't smoke, because this can irritate your mouth and throat.

If you do not have sores in your mouth, you might try eating some sweet or tart foods, such as lemonade; or sucking on hard candy, which can stimulate the production of saliva. Following is a list of other methods to keep your mouth moist as much as possible:

- Suck on ice cubes or cracked ice.
- Take a swallow of your beverage with each bite of food.
- Eat moist foods and drink lots of liquids.
- Try eating cold foods, rather than warm or hot ones.
- Add sauces or syrups, melted butter, gravy, or broth to foods.
- Cookies, breads, and rolls can be "dunked" into tea, coffee, milk, or broth.

Mouth Sores

If you have ever had a canker sore in your mouth, you know how difficult it can be to eat your favorite foods, despite all your efforts to shift the food around to avoid the sore.

Imagine what it is like to eat when you have several of these uncomfortable or even painful sores in your mouth. If you have already experienced this side effect, or are about to have a drug that may induce it, you will be somewhat relieved to know that you can still get nutrition despite this problem, and that the sores *will* go away. In the meantime, your doctor can prescribe medicine to numb the sore area, or he may suggest lozenges or sprays that can numb the area just long enough for you to enjoy your meal.

Avoid such foods as pepper, chili, nutmeg, and other hot spices, and be wary of citrus juices, alcohol, and rough foods. Foods that are acidic or salty can be "toned down" with sugar.

There are a number of foods that are nutritious, tasty, and nonirritating. Many are high in protein as well as calories. Here are some suggestions:

- Milk, milkshakes, malted milks.
- Tea with sugar.
- Prune, apple, pear, and apricot juices.
- High-protein, high-calorie liquid supplements.
- Hot cereals cooked with milk.
- Soft French toast or milk toast.
- Mashed bananas.
- Soft-boiled, lightly scrambled, coddled, or poached eggs.
- Cottage cheese (moisten, if desired, with milk or fruit syrup drained from canned, noncitrus fruit).
- Yogurts.
- Sour cream.
- Gelatin.
- Ice cream.
- Sherbet.
- Watermelon.
- Puddings and custards.
- Fudgesicles and popsicles.
- Applesauce.
- Creamed soups.
- Split-pea soup. ⎫
- Vegetable soup. ⎬ strained; served warm, not hot
- Chicken or beef soup. ⎭
- Mashed or whipped potatoes, thinned with milk or cream.
- Macaroni.
- Rice.
- Ground meat or poultry.
- Baby foods: fruits, vegetables, meats, poultry, and soups.

Make frequent use of a blender or food processor. Cook foods first, then process. Your butcher may be able to grind any meats you especially like. Then cook them slowly and well, as patties or a loaf. If you don't feel like cooking or preparing your own meals, use commercial baby foods, adding a bit of sophisticated flavorings or combining them with canned or frozen soups. You can also use baby foods as the basis for gravy—just add water or milk.

Drinks and soups can be enriched by the addition of eggs. Beat an egg into a milk drink, or drop beaten egg gradually into a soup as it heats in the pot. This makes "egg-drop" soup.

If spoons hurt your mouth, try drinking soups through a straw or from a cup. You might want to try one of the cups intended for tod-dlers—they have covers with a small spout enabling you to direct the liquid away from sore areas.

If you wear dentures and the sores are beneath them, remove the dentures when you eat.

Feeling of Fullness

Many patients complain that they sit down to a meal with enthu-siasm only to feel full before they have eaten much.

Plan to eat smaller, more frequent meals, and be sure each one is nutritious and a good source of calories and protein. Drink liquids *after* you have eaten, so that you are not filled up and bloated even before you begin a meal.

NAUSEA AND EATING

Nausea and eating don't seem to go together—but if you are suf-fering from any degree of queasiness or chronic nausea, because of either chemotherapy or radiation, you still need to maintain your nu-trition status. Your physician may be able to recommend an antinausea medication that will enable you to feel more like eating. Some patients say that marijuana helps.

Be careful to avoid any foods that repel you, even if they were once favorites. If your nausea seems particularly uncomfortable in the early mornings, place melba toast, dry toast, or crackers next to your bed before you go to sleep at night. You will be able to eat them even before you get up in the morning, and this may "settle your stomach." Later you may feel more like eating.

Small, frequent meals will help to keep something in your stomach and prevent nausea, while still giving you nourishment. To minimize tension in your stomach, which exacerbates nausea, try to relax (use relaxation techniques, or ask your doctor for a mild tranquilizer); and eat slowly and chew your food well.

Some people find that drinking liquids at mealtimes, especially coffee and tea, fills their stomach, contributing to nausea. Try drinking any liquids thirty minutes to an hour before or after eating.

Salty foods, rather than sweet ones, are often helpful. Avoid fatty or greasy, fried, overly sweet, spicy, hot, or strong-smelling foods. And *don't* force your favorite foods when you are feeling nauseous, because when you are feeling better, you may find that you have been "turned off" those once-favorites.

Strong food odors may nauseate you, so if possible, let someone else prepare meals, and stay away from the kitchen while he is cooking. Avoid eating in a stuffy, too-warm room or one that is filled with cooking odors or other smells that may be overpowering or disagreeable. Eat in pleasant surroundings—perhaps in your favorite room or chair, with pleasant company, or in front of the television.

Cold-meat plates, sandwiches, fruit plates, cottage cheese, and many other nutritious foods may be more appealing because they have little or no smell. You can make use of convenience foods or take-outs from fast-food restaurants. But avoid going to any restaurants where the smell of a mixture of foods may overwhelm you.

Carbonated beverages, such as cola or ginger ale, help curb nausea. It is often best to first let them stand a bit, opened, to get rid of some of the gas-causing fizz.

Foods that are especially good if you are experiencing nausea are:

- Crackers, dry toast, soda biscuits, plain cookies.
- Carbonated beverages, such as cola or ginger ale.
- Gelatins.
- Tart foods, such as pickles and lemons.
- Sherbets.
- Mildly salty foods, such as pretzels.
- Popsicles.
- Boiled, broiled, or baked chicken (not fried).

Rest after eating, because activity can slow down digestion. If you do want to lie down, keep your head higher than your feet.

Don't be afraid to experiment—some foods that are unappealing to one person may be just fine for another.

Vomiting. Some people feel mildly nauseous after treatment, or remain chronically so, but others become so nauseous they have serious bouts of vomiting. If this happens to you, rinsing your mouth with cool water or mouthwash afterward, and then avoiding all liquids and food until you feel confident that the vomiting has stopped, will help you to feel better.

When vomiting has stopped, try drinking a clear liquid, beginning with just a teaspoonful every ten minutes, gradually increasing the amount and spacing the portions farther apart. The best liquids to try are:

- Carbonated beverages.
- Tea.
- Strained, diluted fruit juices (especially apple, cranberry, grape).
- Clear gelatin.
- Fruit ices (without milk or pieces of fruit).
- Bouillon, clear fat-free broths, consommé.
- Popsicles.

When you find that you are tolerating these, and you no longer feel nauseous, you may want to try "full liquid" (soft) foods, such as cooked cereal, junket, custard, pudding, plain yogurt, eggnog, high-protein diet supplement, ice cream, strained or pureed soups.

If your nausea and vomiting are directly related to a specific treatment, you may find they simply disappear within a certain period. Some people are able to eat their normal foods within a few hours after completion of treatment; others need a few days. But if vomiting persists for more than twenty-four hours, contact your physician.

Diarrhea

Diarrhea may follow radiotherapy or chemotherapy. It may persist for some time or occur only immediately after treatment.

If you are suffering from diarrhea, try going on a clear-liquid diet for one day. Sometimes, allowing the bowels to rest, while replacing body fluids, may correct the problem. Then gradually begin taking full liquids, and finally, meals of more solid food that *exclude* high bulk or roughage (such as bran, whole-grain breads, beans, and skins). All beverages and foods should be warm—neither hot nor cold. These low-fiber foods are good for such a diet:

- Fish, chicken, tender or ground beef.
- Eggs.
- Pureed vegetables.
- Fruit (canned or cooked) without skins.
- Ripe bananas.
- Cooked cereals.
- Smooth peanut butter.

Avoid greasy, fatty, or fried foods, coffee, citrus juices, raw vegetables and fruits (except apples), high-fiber vegetables (such as broccoli, corn, and cauliflower). You may try tea, but it should be very weak.

Diarrhea can cause dehydration and potassium deficiency. Lost fluids can be replaced by drinking lots of clear liquids. Depleted potassium can be replaced by eating bananas, boiled or mashed potatoes, apricot and peach nectar—all of which are rich in potassium but do not cause diarrhea. (Orange juice, saltwater fish, and milk are also high in potassium, but may exacerbate the diarrhea.) If diarrhea persists, call your physician. He may give you an antidiarrhea medication, and perhaps a potassium supplement as well.

Lactose Intolerance

It is possible that your diarrhea has been caused by an intolerance to lactose, a substance found in milk and other dairy products. Symptoms of this condition occasionally follow chemotherapy or radiation that has affected the GI tract.

If your doctor suspects that you have this problem, he may ask you to avoid milk, ice cream, all but natural aged cheeses, instant coffee, cocoa and most chocolate beverages, cream, and desserts with custard or cream filling, because they are all high in lactose.

Some other foods and even medications contain small amounts of lactose, so you may be able to tolerate them only in small quantities. Read all labels carefully. Foods with lactose include breads and baked goods containing milk, gravies with milk, butter, margarine, and yogurt, as well as any prepared products that contain dry milk solids. Many such products are available both with and without milk solids; look for items in your grocery store that are kosher and marked "pareve." They are milk-free. A small *K* in a circle with a *P* underneath may be the only marking, but that should ensure you there is no milk in the product.

Some people who are lactose-intolerant can tolerate buttermilk and yogurt, because these products have been changed during processing. Lact-Aid, a tablet supplying the enzyme lactase (which breaks down lactose) can be added to milk twenty-four hours before use, making it lactose-free but still giving you all the nutritional value of the milk. Mention this to your physician if you suffer from lactose intolerance.

Constipation

Cancer patients often become constipated. Chemotherapy, pain medication, reduced activity, a diet lacking bulk or fluid, intestinal spasms, and emotional stress all can lead to this condition. Exercising as much as you can tolerate—even walking—can be of help. Your doctor may suggest you take a laxative, stool softener, or artificial bulk product. Discuss this with him before taking any of them.

Some high-fiber foods can help. They include:

- Raw fruits and vegetables (leave the skins on).
- Whole-grain breads and cereals.
- Nuts.
- Stewed or dried fruit, such as prunes, apricots, figs, and raisins.
- Brown or wild rice.
- Whole-wheat pasta.
- Unrefined cereal grains.
- Salads.
- Bran.

And drink plenty of liquids (especially hot ones). Prune juice and hot water with lemon juice are particularly good as natural laxatives.

If constipation persists, contact your doctor.

Heartburn. Medications or certain foods may give you heartburn. If so, avoid foods that increase acid output by your stomach. Hot, spicy foods; coffee; and liquor may all cause heartburn. Antacids may help, but if the condition continues, contact your physician.

Diet for Ostomates

Colostomy and ileostomy patients may find that certain foods can cause blockage. These foods include nuts, popcorn, skins on fruit and vegetables, and foods with seeds. Diarrhea is also a common problem, so ostomates should minimize their consumption of raw fruits and vegetables, juices, beer, and spicy foods. Gas-producing foods, such as onions, eggs, fish, and carbonated beverages, may also create a problem.

Urostomy patients are often advised to drink a great deal of clear liquid, to reduce the risk of infection or formation of kidney stones. Many doctors also suggest you include cranberry juice in your regular diet because it keeps urine in an acid state and helps to minimize odors. Generally, you will be able to follow the guidelines for good nutrition, simply remaining alert to some of the potential problems identified here.

Excessive Weight Gain

Some drugs, especially the hormones and cortisone derivatives, contribute to weight gain and water retention. Radiation directed at certain areas of the body can also cause the body to retain water and salt. Of course, a reduction in exercise will also put weight on some people. Those patients who find they can still enjoy all their favorite foods sometimes discover they have grown a size or two.

This is not the time to go on the latest best-selling diet. Discuss your weight gain with your physician. He may suggest a diuretic, but if he says that it is not medically wise to lose weight right now, you may just have to decide to buy or borrow clothes in the next size. More likely, your doctor will suggest some mild exercise, and advise you to limit your salt intake and resist extra goodies like candy and ice cream.

Avoid foods that are high in salt, such as canned soups, herring, sardines, salted crackers, soy sauce, luncheon meats, and potato chips. You can also replace table salt with salt substitutes (available in your supermarket). Read labels on prepared foods to determine their salt content.

Stay away from high-fat foods, too, whenever possible. These include butter, cream, fatty meats, shortening, and nuts.

Too Tired to Eat

That's a common complaint. Treatment can tire you; so can daily trips for radiotherapy. Sometimes, "too tired to eat" really means "too tired to cook."

Let someone else do the work. If family, friends, or neighbors offer to help, let them. You can return the favor later when you feel better. If you can afford it, pay someone to help. Some retired or stay-at-home people are happy to earn extra money preparing home-cooked meals for you to freeze or refrigerate and reheat. Some restaurants (even those that are not take-out places) will prepare main courses and deliver them, or you can arrange for someone to pick them up. Keep frozen dinners on hand.

Many communities have programs that arrange to deliver meals to homebound people. The social worker at your hospital, church or synagogue, community social-service agency, Visiting Nurse Service, or local American Cancer Society may sponsor or be familiar with such programs. Costs are usually nominal.

If you are really too tired to eat, be sure that you are getting enough protein. High-protein snacks may give you fast nourishment as well as energy to eat later.

Vitamin Supplements

Your physician may recommend some vitamin supplements, but it is unlikely that he will prescribe them in large doses. Megavitamins, advocated by some people interested in nutrition, may be harmful to the cancer patient. Taken in excess, certain vitamins, such as A, D, E, and K, may be stored in the liver and cause serious side effects. Do not take any vitamins without first talking to your physician.

Experts in Nutrition

Physicians in some major hospitals and communities specialize in nutrition. If well-trained in this field, they are usually members of the American Society for Clinical Nutrition. Registered dietitians who have been trained in the principles of sound nutrition hold an undergraduate degree, have been certified by the American Dietetic Association, and undergo ongoing education to keep themselves up-to-date on new developments. Both are highly qualified to help you form a nutritional plan.

Qualified nutritionists will have undergraduate, masters, or doctorate degrees in nutrition from an accredited college or university. They will probably be members of the Society for Nutrition Education, the American Institute of Nutrition, or the American Association for Clinical Nutrition. Your local American Cancer Society may be able to recommend a qualified dietitian or nutritionist who can help you.

Beware of people who call themselves nutritionists but have none of the above qualifications.

IF YOU CAN'T EAT ENOUGH

Sometimes all the best efforts of family, friends, dietitians, physicians, and patient are to no avail; you just can't eat enough to maintain satisfactory nutritional status.

There is something you can do about it.

Nutritional supplements and aids. A number of excellent products can be purchased in your drugstore (even occasionally in the supermarket) to enrich your diet. Some come in powder form to be mixed with water, making a high-protein drink. Others are high in calories, with no protein added. There are also high-protein, high-calorie supplements in powder, liquid, and pudding form. While most of these products are only supplements to food, some are complete liquid diets. In addition, there are lactose-free milk substitutes, often high in calories and protein.

The supplements come in both unflavored and a variety of flavored versions. The flavored ones can be consumed just as they are, but the unflavored ones are more suitable for adding to other foods to increase their nutritional value. Some common brands are Citrotein, Controlyte, Ensure, Ensure Plus, Isocal, Isomil, Meritene, Polycose, Sustacal, Sustagen, Carnation Instant Breakfast. Some supplements are available only by prescription. You will need to look carefully at the labels to determine their calorie, protein, and fat content. Consult your physician before using any of them.

These supplements can be used in a number of ways:

- Some can be consumed right out of a can—or can be reconstituted, warmed up, or chilled.
- Some can be poured over cereal, or used instead of water or milk to make hot cereal, omelets, French toast.
- Pudding supplements can be used as dessert toppings, or toppings can be added to them.
- Combine ice cream with liquid supplement to make a nutritious shake.
- Freeze liquid or pudding to make a dessert.
- Add supplement to milk and eggs for an eggnog.
- Blend liquid supplement with fruit, vanilla extract, and cinnamon or sugar to make a shake.
- Mix 12 ounces of supplement with one package of gelatin and ½ cup boiling water to make a gelatin dessert.

Hyperalimentation and tube feedings. Hyperalimentation is the intravenous administration of up to 2,000 calories a day, far more than the amount available in traditional IV bottles, and as much as many people normally consume. In this process, sometimes called *total parenteral nutrition (TPN)*, these nutrients are administered through a catheter in the vein near the neck, *directly* into the superior vena cava, and then into the bloodstream. (The gastrointestinal tract is bypassed.) Or nutrients may be given via a tube inserted through the mouth, nose, or an opening in the esophagus, stomach, or small intestine. This method is called *total enteral nutrition (TEN)*. The nutrients are administered at regular intervals or continuously.

Although hyperalimentation is usually begun in the hospital, it is possible for the patient to continue the procedure at home. Like the right-atrial catheter (discussed in Chapter 6), hyperalimentation allows many cancer patients to have far more freedom of activity while getting the care they need.

Tube feedings are sometimes administered to patients who, because of problems with the throat and esophagus, cannot swallow. For nasogastric feedings, in which a tube is inserted through the nose into the stomach, or gastrostomy feedings, in which the tube is inserted directly into the stomach through the abdomen, nutritious diets of pureed food are used.

Many patients undergoing hyperalimentation or tube feedings are able to go about their daily activities and simply take time to get their feeding while relaxing or watching television. Hyperalimentation may provide all their essential nutrition, or simply supplement the foods they are eating or drinking by normal means. Often it is just a temporary measure until normal eating can be resumed.

Signs of Malnutrition

When you look in the mirror each day, or see a family member daily, it is sometimes difficult to notice loss of weight, particularly if the patient habitually dresses in loose clothes. So use a good bathroom scale to help keep track of weight. In addition to weight loss, other signs of malnutrition include:

- Skin breakdown, such as bedsores.
- Tiredness; desire to stay in bed all day.
- Increasing weakness.
- Irritability.
- Slow healing of any cuts or sores.
- Poor resistance to infections.
- Depression.
- Electrolyte-fluid imbalance, which can lead to: dehydration, edema (swelling), weakness, diminished reflexes, muscle cramps, nausea, diarrhea, impaired mental functioning, seizures, disorientation, and other life-threatening conditions.

Nutrition Can Be Maintained

Cancer patients no longer need to accept malnutrition as an inevitable response to their condition and treatment. If a patient or his family notices that he is becoming malnourished, he can ask the oncologist to recommend an assessment of his nutritional status by a physician who has special training in that field. It is far easier to maintain reasonably good nutrition as a precaution against debilitation than it is to try to rehabilitate someone who is already debilitated.

Sometimes nutritional therapy is initiated in the hospital but neglected when a patient returns home. Be sure that you have been given clear instructions about nutrition before you are discharged, and if not, seek a consultation with a nutritionist or registered dietitian.

CALORIE AND PROTEIN CONTENT

	Amount	Protein (in grams)	Calories
Beverages			
Whole milk	8 oz.	9.0	165
Half-and-half	8 oz.	7.6	330
Buttermilk	8 oz.	8.1	90
Ice-cream soda	12 oz.	2.3	300
Malted milk	12 oz.	13.1	300
Cola	8 oz.	0	105
Fruit punch	8 oz.	0	200
Eggnog	8 oz.	7.8	270
Breads			
Bread	1 slice	2.0	80
Sweet roll	1	3.0	135
Corn bread	1	4.3	136
Vegetables			
Potato	1 small	1.9	68
Beets, carrots, peas, squash	½ cup	approx. 1.0	less than 50
Sugar, Syrups and Jams			
Brown sugar	1 tbsp.	0	51
Cane sugar	1 tbsp.	0	54
Corn syrup	1 tbsp.	0	57
Honey	1 tbsp.	0.1	62
Jams	1 tbsp.	0	55
Maple syrup (pure)	1 tbsp.	0	70
Molasses, cane	1 tbsp.	0	50
Fruits			
Sweetened applesauce	⅓ cup	0.2	100
Banana	1 cup	1.6	136
Fruit cocktail	1 cup	0.4	175
Meats			
Bacon	2 slices	3.6	97
Hamburger	3 oz.	21.8	216
Beef liver	2 oz.	9.0	118
T-bone steak	8 oz.	24.0	235
Roast beef	4 oz.	28.4	300
Frankfurter	1	7.0	124
Baked ham	1 med. slice	31.0	265

CALORIE AND PROTEIN CONTENT

	Amount	Protein (in grams)	Calories
Meat loaf	3 oz.	9.0	316
Roast chicken	4 oz.	30.0	277
Baked fish fillet	4 oz.	30.0	160
Soups			
Pea soup	8 oz.	6.0	245
Cream of mushroom soup	8 oz.	20.0	200
Oyster stew	8 oz.	12.0	200
Potato soup	8 oz.	6.0	215
Eggs			
Boiled in shell	1	6.2	77
Scrambled	1	7.3	106
White only	1	3.4	15
Yolk only	1	2.8	60
Fats and Oils			
Butter	1 tbsp.	0.1	100
Corn oil	1 tbsp.	0	100
Margarine	1 tbsp.	0.1	100
Gravy	½ cup	2.4	400
Desserts			
Puddings	4 oz.	4.5	150
Jell-O	4 oz.	1.6	75
Pie	⅟₇	2.9–9.6	265–350
Ice cream	1 scoop	5.7	295
Cheese cake	3″ × 2″ sq.		300
Chocolate cake	3″ × 2″ sq.	2.2	190
Sponge cake	3″ × 2″ sq.	3.8	117
Brownies (no nuts)	2″ × 2″ sq.	2.0	135
Cookies	1	1.0	55–90
Candies			
Milky Way	1 bar	2.8	284
Hard candy	2 sq.	0	38
Fudge (no nuts)	1 oz.	0.5	115
Cereals and Grains			
Cream of wheat	1 cup	4.5	133
Macaroni	1 cup	6.0	190
Oatmeal	1 cup	5.4	148

CALORIE AND PROTEIN CONTENT

	Amount	Protein (in grams)	Calories
Rice	¾ cup	2.1	103
Spaghetti	1 cup	5.0	155
Condiments and Sauces			
Mayonnaise	1 tbsp.	0.15	92
Peanut butter (creamy)	1 tbsp.	5.2	115
Roquefort dressing	1 tbsp.	0.7	100
Dairy Products			
American cheese	1 slice	7.0	100
Cottage cheese	4 oz.	15.0	110
Heavy cream	1 tbsp.	0.3	50
Sour cream	1 tbsp.	0.8	58
Plain yogurt	8 oz.	8.3	120

Chapter 15

The Team Approach:
Many People Can Help

Nobody ever said cancer was easy. It's not easy to have it, to see someone you care about have it, or to be a health professional who works with patients who have it.

Sometimes it seems lonely. But you don't have to face it alone. Patients, family members, friends, and health professionals all can benefit from the "team approach," which allows you to have continuous caring, helpful support from others.

Your first line of support is your doctor, who is treating you with the goal of curing the disease or significantly extending your life. But in addition to doctors, there are many other professionals whose care and services make it easier for you to cope with cancer. Foremost among them are nurses, including many specialists who work in hospitals, clinics, doctors' offices, through a visiting-nurse program or other home health-care agency. There are also physician's assistants, physical and occupational therapists, speech and hearing therapists, social workers, psychologists, pharmacists, nutritionists, dietitions, technologists, patient representatives in hospitals, health aides and homemakers, volunteers in hospitals and community agencies. You may also use the services of the clergy, and of sympathetic attorneys or financial advisors.

Good hospital care is essential to the cancer patient, but so is good home care, because you may need assistance following hospitalization. Sometimes good home care can even help you avoid hospitalization.

Home-care plans are usually set up by a doctor, nurse, or social worker, and may depend on a referral to a home-care agency based in the hospital itself, in your community, or a privately owned agency. The service or agency often creates the team for you, or simply adds an appropriate health-care professional to the staff already treating you.

Doctors

I have discussed the various kinds of doctors who treat cancer patients, but since doctors are a vital part of the "team approach," the subject deserves further discussion.

Generally speaking, the medical oncologist is the "team leader" for the cancer patient. He monitors all treatment, gives chemotherapy, and refers the patient to other medical specialists whenever necessary.

Radiation oncologists—or radiotherapists, as they are often called—are responsible for radiation therapy. Surgeons or surgical oncologists perform any surgery required. Radiologists will assume responsibility for imaging techniques, often essential to diagnosis and ongoing monitoring of your condition. Many subspecialties of medicine may be represented as consultants; a specialist may even be your primary caregiver. These specialists may be gastroenterologists, pulmonary specialists, or any number of other specialists. Gynecologists and urologists often assume dual roles: surgeon and continued caregiver.

Pain specialists or nutritional specialists may be physicians who are primarily specialists in other areas, with another, related subspecialty.

Psychiatrists can also be helpful to the cancer patient. Some specialize in the relationship between physical disease and emotions; they may even have specific expertise in treating mental and emotional problems that occur in cancer patients. Cancer can cause otherwise mentally healthy patients to exhibit mild to serious emotional upsets. For this reason, some cancer hospitals have a department of psychiatric services, in which psychiatrists, psychologists, and other mental-health professionals offer services to patients. And in general hospitals, psychiatrists often serve as consultants to cancer departments.

Dentists are also an important part of the health team. Frequently they are the first to identify symptoms of oral cancer. They are also able to advise and treat mouth problems that may arise from chemotherapy or from radiation to the head and neck area. The cancer patient should always tell his dentist if he has cancer and is being treated for it. If possible, it is wise to see your dentist prior to beginning treatment.

Nurses

Many nurses specialize in oncology. They work in doctors' offices, clinics, hospitals, and on various home-care teams. No cancer patient's team is complete without them.

Nurses give skilled hands-on care: They draw blood, administer medications orally or by injection, give catheter and other kinds of tube care; they care for surgical wounds, stomas, and bed sores; in short, they deal with countless physical and medical needs. Nurses have an important role as teachers, too, instructing patients in self-care and showing families how to care for the patient. Perhaps more than any other profession, nursing offers dedicated men and women an opportunity to give a variety of compassionate and intellectually stimulating care to patients, both directly and indirectly.

Depending on the laws of your state and on the rules in the hospital where you are treated, nursing responsibilities vary. Nurses are educated at various levels. They may be graduates of a nursing school and hence have the letters R.N. following their name, denoting that they are licensed by the state as professional registered nurses. A great number of nurses are graduates of college as well as nursing school, and have a bachelor's degree in science along with a nursing degree. Other nurses have chosen to have additional training and specialize, perhaps in oncology or stoma care. There are almost thirty different specialty associations of professional nurses in the United States; Canadian nurses also have a number of specialties. To retain their licenses, in some states, R.N.'s are required to enroll in continuing-education programs. A substantial number of nurses pursue still further rigorous academic training and receive a master's or doctorate degree in nursing.

Licensed practical nurses have less formal education in nursing than do R.N.'s. They are equipped to take care of patients with simpler needs, requiring only routine treatment and care. These nurses work in many settings, usually under the direct supervision of a registered nurse. L.P.N.'s are licensed in most states; they are excellent and important caregivers.

But none of the above really shows how important the nurse's role is. In hospitals, each nurse is there for eight hours a day (sometimes longer), serving the emotional and physical needs of patients. They also serve as the eyes and ears of the physician, making important decisions as to when a patient needs to see a doctor immediately.

In offices or clinics where radiation or chemotherapy is administered, nurses assume responsibility for much direct patient care, education, and recordkeeping.

Nurses are, in short, indispensable.

Physician's Assistants

Physician's assistants, known as P.A.'s, are trained in certain aspects of the practice of medicine to provide assistance to a physician. They practice under the direction and supervision of a physician. Training programs vary in length from a few months to two years. They work in doctors' offices, in clinics, and in hospitals, and do a great deal of hands-on care. In many instances, and in some states they are permitted to write prescriptions, and they perform many routine medical tasks for the doctor who supervises them. They often give chemotherapy.

Although it is still a fairly new profession, as compared to nursing, P.A.'s play an important role in surgical and medical care, including that of cancer patients. Their national organization is the American Association of Physician's Assistants (AAPA).

Physical Therapists

Physical therapists assist in the examination, testing, and treatment of people who are temporarily or permanently physically disabled. They are an important part of the team for cancer patients whose disease or treatment has in some way limited their movement. Physical therapists use special exercises, applications of heat or cold, sonar waves, and other techniques. They work in hospitals, nursing homes, and on home-care teams. Some have their own offices, treating people who have been referred to them by physicians.

Physical therapists are very helpful to postmastectomy patients in particular, and to anyone else whose treatment has affected muscle tone, coordination, and strength. They often begin by teaching and helping patients to do "range-of-motion" exercises and to perform some simple self-care activities in a hospital bed. Goals vary according to the physical potential and age of the patient, but a return to functioning as normally as possible is always utmost in the therapist's mind.

Occupational Therapists

Occupational therapists use purposeful specific activity with people whose ability to function independently is limited for any number of reasons, including physical injury or illness. Cancer patients whose ability to function may have been disrupted are often helped to learn alternative ways to achieve and maintain independence. For instance, a patient who is wheelchair-bound can learn to dress and cook. Occupational therapists work in hospitals and other institutions, and are often part of the home-care team.

In any of these settings, O.T.'s try to help you do as much for yourself as possible. Often they accomplish this with the aid of various equipment, ranging from simple devices that aid in eating, dressing, or reaching, to special chairs (wheel or stationary), beds, or bathroom safety and convenience aids. The therapist can arrange for you to obtain these items, usually from a local medical-equipment store or large pharmacy. Much of this equipment is reimbursed completely or in part by Medicare or medical-insurance companies. The supplier can usually advise you about this reimbursment.

Speech and Hearing Therapists

Sometimes called speech and hearing pathologists, these professionals are trained to treat people with communication disorders. Cancer patients who have had head or neck surgery are often in need of these professionals to help them regain the ability to speak. These therapists can also recommend and help you obtain any needed equipment, much of which is paid for by insurance.

Technologists

Technologists, or technicians, work in many medical settings. They usually work under the supervision of doctors and/or nurses, doing such diverse things as drawing blood in the office or hospital, taking X rays and electrocardiograms. Many technologists are highly trained, especially those who work with some of the newer nuclear imagery equipment. Technologists are important members of the health-care team.

Social Workers

Social workers are perhaps best described as "problem solvers." Their skills are diverse and, depending on the setting in which they work, are used in different ways. Generally, they work to enhance the relationships between individuals and their environment or surroundings.

Medical social workers, especially those who work with cancer patients, are familiar with the physical and psychological aspects of cancer. They are sensitive to the social factors that influence the way each patient may react to his disease, and the way other people react to him. They are trained to provide short-term or even intensive long-term counseling and psychotherapy for individuals and groups. Social workers often coordinate resources, initiate and supervise home-care services, or refer patients and families to those community agencies that offer this help.

In Chapter 16, I'll discuss the emotional reactions to cancer and how social workers help patients cope.

To be a member of the Academy of Certified Social Workers and (in most states) to become a certified or licensed social worker, a person must have a master's degree in social work from an accredited graduate school of social work and pass a certification or licensing test. Many social workers, especially those who direct departments of social work or who teach in schools of social work, have earned a doctorate in the field.

Social workers with an undergraduate degree in social work are also on staff in many hospitals and health-maintenance organizations (HMOs). "Social-work aides" are often people with good on-the-job training and a commitment to helping people. These professionals usually do not counsel patients, except under close supervision; instead, they help them to obtain needed services and/or equipment.

Social workers at every level of education are involved in the discharge planning of patients, ensuring that the patient will get any needed services at home.

Psychologists

Psychologists have a master's degree or doctorate in psychology, and must pass a test to be licensed in the state in which they practice.

There are many types of psychologists, reflecting the kinds of work they do. Clinical psychologists are those most likely to work with cancer patients. They offer counseling and short- or long-term psychotherapy in hospital or private settings. Their techniques are similar to those offered by social workers, but psychologists usually are not involved in referrals to such services as home care. Since hospitals often maintain departments of social-work services, psychologists are more likely to be found in private practices, or attached to the psychiatry department in a hospital. Many psychologists have made a specialty of working with cancer patients, using a variety of techniques. Those with doctorates in clinical psychology are highly trained.

Pharmacists

Pharmacists have intensive, ongoing training in the preparation and dispensation of medications. Some pharmacists, especially those who work in hospital pharmacies, are specially trained in the effects of chemotherapy and in administration of pain medication. They work closely with oncologists.

In choosing a pharmacy for your medication needs at home, find one that takes a complete drug history from you and then keeps track of all the drugs, prescription and nonprescription, that you use. Many pharmacies now have computers so that they can efficiently maintain your medication profile. In this way, they can make sure that you are using your drugs correctly and that there is no risk of a harmful interaction between them.

Pharmacists are also a good source of information about side effects and symptoms that should be reported to your physician, interactions with drugs and food, proper timing of doses, and special storage requirements. They can even help you complete insurance forms if you have coverge for drugs.

Before leaving the hospital, you may wish to have the hospital pharmacist get in touch with your neighborhood pharmacist, or vice versa. Give each the other's name and phone number.

Nutritionists and Dietitians

As discussed in Chapter 14, nutrition is essential in the treatment of, and recovery from, cancer. Sometimes a specialist's help is required. Registered dietitians hold an undergraduate degree, have been trained in the principles of sound nutrition, and are certified by the American Dietetic Association. Nutritionists who hold an undergraduate or graduate degree in nutrition are usually members of one of the major nutrition associations. Many of them are specially trained and prepared to help you with a good nutrition plan at home as well as in the hospital.

If you want to consult a dietitian, please be sure to read Chapter 14 first; then ask your physician, or another respected professional, to recommend one to you. Be sure to check the qualifications of anyone who calls himself a nutritionist, since many have simply designated the title upon themselves.

Respiratory Therapists

Respiratory therapists are important health-care workers in the hospital. They help patients who have breathing difficulties to restore, improve, or maintain lung function. After surgery, the respiration therapist may visit you to teach you deep-breathing exercises, followed by coughing. This helps to avoid the accumulation of mucus in the lungs, which can lead to pneumonia and other complications. Registered respiration therapists use and maintain various types of machines from simple nebulizers, a device that produces a spray and also administers medication, to complex ventilators that help patients take in oxygen and exhale carbon dioxide.

Patient Representatives

Many hospitals have a department with trained personnel called patient representatives, ombudsmen, or patient advocates. Generally they are available to all patients. They serve as concerned representatives of patients and their families, explain hospital policies and procedures, refer patients to appropriate services, often provide notary-public and interpreter services, and help patients and their families with problems that other staff have not been able to resolve. They often respond directly to verbal and written inquiries, suggestions and complaints regarding problems with patient services, and then follow through to determine that solutions have been reached.

Patient representatives are truly the troubleshooters of the hospital, and although they are paid by the hospital, they are the patients' advocates. They have a strong code of ethics, and maintain patient confidentiality. Someone from their department, or a designated representative, is often on call twenty-four hours a day.

Discharge Planners

Most hospitals have someone who helps to make plans for patients to leave the hospital. Ideally, a health-care professional such as a nurse or social worker assumes this responsibility, but this is not always the case. In some hospitals, the discharge planner is someone with good administrative skills but without patient-care background.

Before leaving the hospial, you should feel certain that you will be able to manage safely, and that your condition will not deteriorate because of a lack of some needed services, such as someone to bring you meals, help you bathe and dress if you cannot do those things alone.

Hospitals may not be paid by Medicare or other medical-insurance companies when a patient stays in the hospital longer than is typical for a given illness or surgical procedure, or when you no longer require skilled care. Thus, hospitals sometimes seem to be in a hurry to discharge you—and it is the discharge planners' responsibility to be sure that you are ready to go home.

Speak up if you feel that you are being discharged before you are ready; your doctor, a social worker, or a patient representative may be able to work with the discharge planner to help you get the services you need.

Home Health Aides and Homemakers

A home health aid or homemaker can play the crucial role in a patient's being able to be in his own home safely and comfortably after or during cancer treatment.

Home care in itself deals with a wide range of services, including skilled nursing, nutritional services, and various therapies, as well as less skilled personnel for homemaking and personal care, such as bathing, dressing, eating, taking one's temperature, changing bandages, and doing exercises.

Some of this important care can be performed by homemakers and home health aides. The exact titles for these people vary, depending on local practice: Those who perform household duties are often called homemakers, housekeepers, or home helps. Those who perform personal-care services may be called nursing assistants, health aides, home health aides, orderlies, or attendants. These aides should have at least sixty hours of training as recommended by the National HomeCaring Council.

Home aides can be found through home health employment agencies, which, it is hoped, have checked out their references carefully and given them a written examination. Many aides will also perform some light household duties, such as shopping, cooking, and laundry. They will help you with all personal care and any activities of your daily life, as well as accompanying you to the physician. Agencies that provide aides often also provide regular visits from an R.N. to ensure that optimum care is being given.

The social worker, nurse, or discharge planner at the hospital can usually find you a good home health agency to provide you with this help.

Medicare and other insurance companies will sometimes pay for a part-time aide, or contribute toward a full-time one. Community social-service agencies will also sometimes provide financial assistance. The American Cancer Society may be able to direct you toward this help.

Clergy

The clergy of all faiths are usually caring, compassionate people who know how to be quiet, involved listeners, and to convey to patients and their families that God is always with them, ready to hear their fears, anxieties, and to support them with His mercy.

Clergy often visit their congregants when they are ill in the hospital or at home, and will bring word to their congregation when one of their members is ill. The congregation will often respond with acts of kindness—cards, flowers, visits, and help for the patient or loved ones at home.

Many hospitals have chaplains of various denominations on staff. They may conduct regular services in a chapel or some other area set aside for that purpose. In addition, chaplains will make rounds in the hospital, visiting patients whom they have already met, and becoming acquainted with those who seem to be in need of religious comfort.

In many hospitals, chaplains serve on various committees, such as those that work to protect patients' rights or uphold medical ethics. In some hospitals, the chaplains work along with physicians, nurses, and social workers on discharge planning, making sure that the patient will be able to function safely at home and have all his needs met by family, friends, or outside help.

If you are religiously observant, a visit by a chaplain of your faith can be very reassuring and comforting. It may lead to a close bond that is very meaningful to you. Even if you have not previously demonstrated any interest in formal religion, you may welcome a visit from a chaplain of your own or another denomination. Clergy who are interested in working with cancer patients usually have had some special training in the field, and so can be enormously helpful. If clergy are not on staff at your hospital, and you are not near your home or do not have a spiritual leader, tell the nurse you want to see a chaplain (minister or rabbi). All hospitals have some referral service to meet this need.

Volunteers

Volunteers in hospitals or in outpatient programs, such as those sponsored by the American Cancer Society, assist with many services that are not provided by anyone else in the community. In some hospitals the volunteers escort patients to their rooms; deliver a newspaper, book, or gift; and make periodic friendly visits.

Such programs have been praised by many health professionals, for although these volunteer visitors may be without formal credentials, they are often people who have themselves had cancer, and they bring a measure of understanding and empathy that many professionals cannot. They also serve as role models. Because they have had cancer, are functioning well and have perhaps even made a recovery, they can give a patient the real hope that he, too, will soon be up and about. And they can give many tips on living a good, full life despite serious illness or disability.

Often this friendly, nonclinical visit can help you start to talk about fears and concerns that you have not discussed with doctors, nurses, or social workers. You may then choose to explore these feelings with professionals.

Volunteers can also do many tasks for a patient that no one else does: write a letter to out-of-town family or friends, pick up some magazines or a favorite cologne, and—perhaps just as important—bring a little bit of the "outside world" to a hospitalized or homebound patient. Sometimes the visitor's description of the holiday decorations downtown, or a detailed account of a good movie, or help in picking out gifts for a favorite niece or nephew from a current catalog, can do more to raise your spirits than all the psychiatrists, social workers, and antidepressant medications put together. Volunteers are usually trained to maintain patient confidentiality, and are often supervised by social workers.

In the community, volunteers often help arrange transportation and escort services to take cancer patients for treatments. They may work in a Meals On Wheels program, delivering nutritious meals to the homes of those unable to prepare or obtain their own meals, help care for children of patients, or meet any number of other patient needs. Some programs of the American Cancer Society help out with these needs; often churches, synagogues, and other religiously related community social-service groups—as well as the American Red Cross, United Way, United Fund, and Community Chest—provide such services.

Patient-Account or Finances Department

Hospitals usually have a department called Patient Account or Patient Finances. That department is responsible for collecting money for all services offered at the hospital.

Usually, people who work with these departments are compassionate people and will listen carefully to anyone who offers a reasonable excuse for not paying a bill. Often they will allow you to pay it in installments; or if you simply have no funds, they will help you to apply for government aid, such as Medicaid. They will work carefully with your insurance company, and unless you have no insurance, or the company has refused to pay the hospital, they are unlikely to ask for the entire cost of the hospital stay.

If you feel a bill is incorrect, or if you simply cannot pay it, call or stop by the finances department and try to make satisfactory arrangements for payment. If you cannot resolve it yourself, ask a patient representative or social worker for assistance.

If your concern is with the physician's bill or bills, discuss it first with his office manager or whoever takes care of the billing. If the problem is not resolved to your satisfaction, discuss it with the physician himself.

Any of these people just mentioned may be able to guide you towards getting good care even if you can't pay for it.

Paying the bills when you can't. Cancer can be expensive, but no one in the United States or Canada needs to go without treatment because they can't afford it. Neoplastic or oncology clinics in major hospitals are usually directed by experienced oncologists who supervise and train the younger doctors, who, along with dedicated nurses, will often provide you with more comprehensive care than you can get in the private offices of noncancer specialists. Clinics will usually accept whatever insurance you have, guide you toward seeking Medicaid, or accept fees on a sliding scale based on ability to pay.

Veterans of the Armed Forces are eligible for care in a veteran's hospital, most of which also maintain outpatient clinics for both general and specialty care.

Medicare is an insurance program administered by the Health Care Financing Administration of the federal government. It is for people over sixty-five years of age and those who have been disabled for two years or more. Cancer can sometimes be considered a disability, making you eligible for Medicare.

Medicare is an entitlement program, available to everyone who meets certain criteria, but it is not means-tested (a millionaire is entitled to it just as much as someone who is very poor). Your local social-security office can give you full details about application and coverage.

Medicaid is a program that offers assistance to low-income patients. It helps pay for a number of different kinds of health care. Eligibility is means-tested, based on income and financial resources, including savings, property, and other income-yielding resources.

Medicaid is not uniform throughout the country, because it is paid for in large part by state and local governments, along with the federal government. Your hospital may be able to advise you on application and coverage. Or contact your local department of human services. The local social-security office may also be able to tell you where to apply.

Inability to obtain insurance. If you have insurance, *keep it*. It may be very difficult to get insurance if you don't already have it. If you have a job, don't leave it until you fully explore all conversion options. If you are unable to obtain insurance through a job, private or group insurance plans, Health Maintenance Organization, Medicare, or Medicaid, and you feel that in some way you have been unfairly treated by an insurance company, contact your state department of insurance. If you have been denied disability through the Social Security Administration or Medicaid, you can appeal the decision. You must file a request for reconsideration with the appropriate agency, and you can usually be represented by a lawyer if you so desire. For further information, contact your local social-security office, the local department of human services, or a legal-aid society in your community. A social worker at the hospital or in a community agency, or someone in the patient accounts department at the hospital, may also be able to give you information on the procedure.

Attorneys

It's a good idea to have an attorney; a good one is like a trusted friend who can help you put things in order, and thus give you a certain peace of mind. If you don't have a lawyer, ask friends for a recommendation, or call the local bar association; they can give you the names and phone numbers of lawyers in your area.

Job discrimination. Many employers are reluctant to hire people who have been treated for cancer; or if you develop cancer, an employer may try to "ease you out." The law is on your side (The Rehabilitation Act of 1973: Sections 503, 504), but you may still be uncomfortable with more subtle forms of discrimination. However, the law is clear, and if you feel you are being discriminated against because of cancer, in looking for a job or on the job, you should discuss this with an attorney. You can also contact your local American Cancer Society division, which may be able to give you specific information on state and local laws and provide you with a list of those who can help you (although the ACS does not represent patients in any legal action).

Providing for loved ones. Everyone should have a last will and testament. Even if you don't have much in the way of money, property, and assets, whatever you do have should be distributed to your loved ones as you wish. If someone dies without a will, the government will decide "who gets what," and taxes may be considerably higher.

You don't have to have cancer to realize you should have a will, but the cancer patient, more than anyone else, is aware that no one lives forever.

Power of attorney. This may be the time to consider giving a trusted relative or friend the power of attorney to sign checks for you, or to make any important decisions for you in the event that you become unable to do so.

Financial Advisers

Whether you have a limited amount of savings or a considerable amount of regular income, a financial adviser can counsel you on the best ways to invest or organize your money to pay for any anticipated or unanticipated expenses you may incur during your illness.

Your bank or a brokerage firm may be able to recommend a financial adviser. This is probably not the time to take financial risks; be sure that the counselor you choose has a sound reputation. You might wish to consult an attorney as well.

Chapter 16
Emotional Reactions and Stress

Cancer has a tremendous emotional impact on patients, their families and friends. From the time of diagnosis throughout the treatment process, life is seldom just as it was before.

Reactions to diagnosis vary, and are not always directly related to the severity of the disease or the prognosis. Many people with curable cancers become depressed, and some with diseases that are highly resistant to treatment maintain an optimistic attitude.

It is normal for a patient to feel any number of mixed emotions, especially at time of diagnosis. Some people initially cope with the news they have cancer by appearing not to cope at all. They may become angry, lashing out at everyone, or they may seem not to have even heard anything, as if denial will cancel out the truth. Often they are unable to sleep or eat, or they may have difficulty in concentrating or working.

If your diagnostic workup took a while to complete, you may have had some time to get used to the idea that cancer was a possibility, and so the final diagnosis might not be an overwhelming surprise. On the other hand, if the diagnosis was made during routine medical tests, you may be in a state of shock, and it may take longer for the news to sink in.

However you react to the news that you have cancer, in time you will probably accept the information and may even go about your usual activities while receiving treatment. You may have many difficult times but still manage to function adequately.

The range of emotional reaction can perhaps best be illustrated in the words of two forty-five-year-old women who both had breast cancer with a favorable prognosis, and had similar prediagnosis life-styles.

One patient said:

I know it sounds corny, but somehow the sun seems brighter and the grass seems greener these days. I always loved to walk in the park near our house, but often I was too busy to find time. Now I still have the same job and home obligations, but I find time to walk in the park almost every day. I know they haven't done any landscaping there recently, but every tree and little bush looks more beautiful than ever. I enjoy watching the seasons change, treasuring each one, but also looking forward to the next.

A postcard or phone call from a friend I haven't seen for a while seems very precious. I guess you might say life suddenly seems sweeter now that I know it's no longer guaranteed.

Lest you think I'm some kind of saint, you should know that I have terrible crying jags at times, get into loud arguments with my husband, and drive the kids crazy about keeping their rooms neat.

The other patient said:

I'm having trouble getting it together. So many things I used to enjoy just have no meaning anymore. I always loved to browse in bookstores, buying a book or two to read at night curled up by the fire. Sometimes I would buy one to put away for vacation time. But now I have trouble concentrating and I'm scared to plan *anything* that relates to the future.

I shrink from friends who want to make plans for a few weeks hence, even though my doctor assures me I'm doing nicely.

I go wherever my husband, the kids, or our friends suggest, but I'm sure I'm pretty poor company. I feel and show no enthusiasm, and my kids are a bit puzzled now that I never bother them to clean up their rooms.

The first woman is coping well. She has focused on the "positives," feeling she didn't live life to its fullest when she took good health for granted. At times she is full of self-pity and anger about her disease, and she takes out this anger on those she loves. But she has not changed from a pleasant, outgoing person into a self-pitying, angry woman.

The second woman may not alarm people. She doesn't complain, she doesn't snap at the kids, and although she doesn't show any enthusiasm, she goes along with the crowd. But she sounds depressed, doesn't she?

If someone suggested that she see a counselor or join a self-help group, she might respond by saying, "Why? What can they do for me? I've got cancer, so of course I'm depressed. When the doctor tells me I'm better, then I'll begin to enjoy life again. Meantime, just leave me alone." This kind of reaction—sometimes expressing itself as an empty feeling, inertia, or lack of goals—is a sign of mild depression. Like feelings of anger, guilt, and resentment, it is understandable. But if such reactions begin to interfere with your life or the lives of those you care about, it is wise to do something about them.

Coping Better

When asked how they are doing, many cancer patients will say that they are hanging in there, but they're not quite sure how they are doing it. Learning that other patients are struggling to cope with the feelings that cancer evokes can be enormously helpful to them. Many read books by cancer patients about their experience with the disease; others spend hours in the library reading medical journals on the subject.

A number of people find they do best by seeking and accepting active treatment, while still denying or minimizing the seriousness of their disease. One patient persisted in saying, "I have just a touch of cancer." Such people often plan vacations, job-related goals, and other activities far in advance, as if to say, "Of course I'll be fine." However, if a medical setback occurs, they may be more devastated than the patient who is more realistic and has guarded optimism.

Another patient copes by setting limited goals: planning a vacation a month, rather than a year, in advance; choosing to repair the lamp in one room rather than changing the light fixtures throughout the house; or planning to submit a still-life photograph—instead of a series of sports photos—to the company's art show.

Some patients develop a sense of mastery over their illness by learning self-care, keeping accurate records of treatment and meals, or doing some volunteer work that allows them to help others.

There are many ways of coping, some helpful, some not so.

Those who cope well do some of these things:

- assimilate the impact of the diagnosis gradually, allowing time to gather together their thoughts and devise reasonable ways of handling the situation.
- seek appropriate medical care.
- share their concerns openly with family and close friends.
- strike a balance between independence and dependence:
  They enlist help from friends and family when they need it, but do as much for themselves as possible.
- maintain hope, but do not deceive themselves.
- set priorities; if energy is limited, they do what is most important to them.

- seek information to better understand their condition, but at the same time occasionally rely on defense mechanisms: repression (unconscious forgetting) or avoidance (conscious decision not to hear what they don't want to hear) of information that may create anxiety.
- maintain self-esteem by remembering that they are still the same people they were before they developed cancer.
- give some thought—without dwelling on it—to preparation for anything that may occur.
- maintain control over their lives; in some instances by learning certain illness-related procedures, such as ostomy or catheter care.
- set attainable, limited goals.
- make use of available emotional-support resources, such as individual or group counseling.
- maintain religious faith.

Those who do not cope as well often:

- repress their feelings.
- feel great anger, which is often turned inward to become depression.
- feel that cancer has been a tremendous assault to their sense of control, self-esteem, and independence.
- refuse to speak to others or seek counseling about their feelings.
- are submissive and withdrawn.
- blame themselves or others for their disease.
- continually displace their emotions onto other people. For instance, patients may be fearful of showing anger to the doctor or nurse, so instead become angry with their family.
- frequently project their feelings onto others. For instance, a patient may be envious of a family member who is well enough to play golf, but claim that the family member is envious of him for getting so much attention.
- have magical expectations that everything will be all right with *or* without treatment.
- regress to such an early stage of emotional development that they become an unnecessary burden on others.
- deny illness to the extent that treatment is abandoned or never sought.
- continue, well past initial diagnosis, to say, "Why me?"
- refuse all intimacy with loved ones.

The list of ways to cope or not cope is endless; hopefully, you will find a way that works for you. But most of those who cope successfully realize that they need help from others.

When Help Is Needed

A good rule of thumb is: If you think you would like some help in coping with cancer, then you need it. It is sensible to seek individual or group counseling if you feel you need to hear about how others are coping, or want someone to confide in, or feel that you are burdening family and friends with your problems. I will discuss the kinds of help available later on in this chapter.

You should seek help if you are finding that emotions or stress are interfering with your life in such a way that you are not functioning a good deal of the time. Anyone who shows the following symptoms of depression should be evaluated by an experienced mental-health professional:

- Exaggerated feelings of sadness, melancholy, despair, and discouragement.
- Inability to eat, not related to treatment or disease.
- Sleep disorders (inability to sleep, or sleeping too much).
- Total social withdrawal.
- Frequent crying.
- Feelings of hopelessness, and brooding about the past.
- Excessive anger or irritability.
- Exaggerated fears of inadequacy and worthlessness.
- Inability to concentrate on anything at home, school, or work.
- Little or no interest in activities that used to be pleasurable.
- Far less energy than is normal under circumstances of illness or treatment.
- Loss of all interest in, or enjoyment of, sex and intimacy.
- A general slowing down of speech, thoughts, or actions.

Other warning signs that may require psychological intervention include panic or anxiety attacks. These attacks may be unrelated to treatment, and usually come on with an intense, overwhelming wave of fear and anxiety. Such attacks are often accompanied by shortness of breath, palpitations, pain or discomfort in chest, choking or smothering sensations, dizziness, feelings of unreality, tingling in hands or feet, hot and cold flashes, sweating, faintness, trembling or shaking. Awaiting a biopsy report would certainly be reasonable cause for a surge of panic and is no great cause for alarm. However, if these attacks occur with any regularity or seem to have no direct cause, and if your physician has ruled out any medical cause for these symptoms, the situation should be brought to the attention of an experienced mental-health professional.

Denial, anger, and guilt all serve a healthy purpose at some time or other, but in cancer patients they can interfere with receiving appropriate and recommended medical care. For instance, a patient who denies his illness may become careless about following the doctor's orders. An angry patient may resent the doctor's authority and control over his life and so refuse to cooperate. And someone who feels guilty for getting sick may choose to punish himself more by ignoring the doctor's recommendations and hence reducing his chance for successful treatment.

Such patients should receive some form of counseling. Other concerns can sometimes be addressed without this help, just by being aware of the problem.

Altered Body Image

Cancer treatment, and cancer itself, can change your appearance. As discussed earlier, side effects of chemotherapy can cause hair loss and changes in weight distribution; and many surgical procedures change bodily appearance and function.

But often one's appearance is not significantly changed, or the changes may not be apparent to others. A woman with a good wig can look every bit as attractive as she did before her hair loss; a man with a colostomy can be dressed as fashionably as before. But this is of little consolation if you look different to yourself or feel you look different to others.

This feeling that you are changed and different is particularly pronounced in women who have had a mastectomy. Despite a natural-looking prosthesis and well-fitting clothes, some women never feel as feminine and attractive as they felt prior to surgery.

Many patients simply need time to adjust to their changed body. Others find that these changes continue to adversely affect their self-esteem long after surgery or treatment. Reassurances from family and friends can do a great deal to restore confidence in yourself, but many people are helped most by various self-help groups in which they meet other people who have gone through or are going through the same changes.

Feeling that you are no longer attractive or desirable is not unusual, but if such emotions do not diminish in time, you should seek help.

Change in Family Roles

When one member of a family is ill, the relationships in a family often change. The financial provider may no longer work, the person responsible for cooking or driving the children to school may be unable to do so, or a grandmother may "drop everything" to care for the children. A ripple effect can take place when a dependent person is catapulted into a role of responsibility, or when an independent head of a family relinquishes that role.

If you no longer can perform some or all of your former tasks you may feel depressed and worthless. Many family members would rather not have to assume new responsibilities, some take it in their stride, and a few may become bossy in their new role.

Changes in roles can occur suddenly or develop gradually over a period of time. Family members who remain sensitive to underlying meanings may be able to minimize the emotional impact. For instance, people who can no longer shop or cook may still feel they maintain control over the kitchen if they can plan the meals, make out the marketing list, and provide recipes. Those who can no longer go to work and bring home a paycheck can still do much of the family budgeting and find useful tasks to do at home.

You and your family will cope best with these changes if you realize that *you* haven't changed but are just performing new and different jobs.

Sexual Concerns

Many cancer patients have concerns about sexual performance; others lose interest in sex. Either situation can cause a problem if the patient's partner retains interest and desire. And on top of these problems, despite all information to the contrary, many cancer patients hesitate to engage in sex because they're afraid of transmitting the disease to their partners.

Unfortunately, most oncologists do not initiate discussions about sex, yet studies show that most patients wish their doctors would do so. Other health professionals, such as nurses, social workers, and psychiatrists, are more likely to bring it up, but not all patients have substantial contact with these professionals. Too often, doctors fail to help patients with this important quality-of-life issue, as if it were unrelated to the illness or treatment. This is not always a fair assumption, and many patients require some education and support from professionals who can discuss these concerns in a comfortable, natural way.

Those patients for whom treatment affects sexual performance need specific help in learning new coital techniques and alternative ways of sexual expression. Certain treatments for female genital cancers damage the genitals or the vaginal passage, making intercourse painful, difficult, or impossible. Surgery for male urinary cancers, ostomies, and spinal-cord injuries can destroy nerves and lead to partial or total impotence. Despite these problems, sexual expression and/or intercourse is not necessarily precluded, but the psychological impact on both patient and partner can keep them from even trying.

Sexual difficulties and decreased desire can also be caused by fatigue from treatment or from the disease itself. Premature menopausal symptoms in women undergoing chemotherapy can also cause temporary problems. Chemotherapy, radiation, or surgery for testicular cancer and some other urological cancers can render a man sterile. For this reason, men may choose to bank their sperm prior to treatment.

But psychological concerns, rather than physical disability, are the most frequent cause of sexual disorders in cancer patients. Anxiety and depression concerning diagnosis and outcome, fear of inability to function, and a change in self-image can all contribute to the problem. Patients who have had mastectomies or head-and-neck surgery resulting in marked cosmetic changes are especially vulnerable to feeling undesirable. Partners are not always supportive; changes in appearance *can* be a "turn-off" for some people. And patients who are lonely and do not have a partner at all may feel hopeless about ever being loved.

Issues of self-esteem are perhaps the greatest roadblock to sexual expression; those who feel threatened by the disease itself, the treatment results, or impaired functioning at work or home often lose interest in sex.

The cancer patient's partner can be a great source of comfort in reassuring the patient that he or she is still desirable and attractive, but this caring and support can sometimes backfire. The man who feels his wife has been through so much following her mastectomy may hesitate to approach her sexually out of fear of physically hurting her, or of sapping her energy. She, in turn, may misinterpret this caution as disinterest. Or a wife who has become unusually maternal in her approach to caring for her husband during his treatment may begin to see him as somehow "emasculated." Loving as she may be, she no longer sees him as the same strong sexual partner she remembers from his precancer days. In response to this new motherly, nurturant personality, he may find her less sexually desirable than she was before he became sick. Throughout treatment, it is very important to discuss all such feelings and fears lovingly and honestly with your partner. Your relationship—and your recovery—can only benefit from such openness.

Patients who have no regular sexual partner often hesitate to begin new relations, feeling that they are no longer attractive or able to function normally. (It may be reassuring for you to know that many people with a history of cancer, including those who have had mastectomies or other surgical procedures that change appearances, have gone on to form new and lasting relationships and to raise families.)

Many sexual problems that do occur are the result of people's assumption that all sexual contact must result in intercourse and orgasm. Although sex educators tell us that sex is far more than intercourse, that has been the only form of sexual expression for many people. Some books about sex are listed in Appendix VII, and they are very helpful in pointing out the many ways of expressing sexuality.

Cancer does not have to be the end of intimacy or sexuality; many patients say that feelings of closeness and warmth have increased during this time, even if intercourse itself is less frequent.

Sex counselors can be helpful (many hospitals have departments of sexuality, where trained professionals can be consulted). Your doctor, nurse, or a medical social worker at the hospital should be able to refer you to one if you would like professional help in this area.

Fear of Recurrence

Some patients say that the fear of cancer recurrence never fully leaves them. Every ache, pain, and discomfort sets off a chain of questions and concerns, all of which center on the big question: Is this a recurrence or spread of my cancer?

It is difficult for the patient with a history of cancer to strike a good balance between careful self-monitoring and cancer phobia. Ideally, you will have regular checkups with a medical oncologist and call him between visits if you have any symptoms that could be related to cancer. You will not ignore anything that could indicate a spread to the bones or lungs, but you will not get hysterical each time you have a cold, virus, or sore back.

Yet recurrence is a natural concern, especially for patients who have known other people who suffered a recurrence years after they were initially treated and pronounced well.

Even if you have completed treatment and view yourself as a survivor, you may feel changed. You may feel victorious and have an extra zest for life, or you may never fully regain your sense of self-esteem. Some people continually find it difficult to plan ahead. Role reversals or shifts in family relationships that took place during treatment may remain. Even if you return to your former activities, you may never really feel the same.

One organization, called CHUMS (Cancer Hopefuls United for Mutual Support—which has chapters throughout the country; see Appendix V), addresses many of the issues of those survivors: people who are receiving treatment or have a history of cancer. They maintain their optimistic outlook, even though they admit that their fear of recurrence lingers for years.

It is useful to maintain some concern about recurrence, because it keeps you going back for checkups. But if that concern takes precedence in your life over all else, interfering with your enjoyment of present health, it can become destructive.

If you do have a recurrence, it often has a greater psychological impact than the original diagnosis did. Your defenses may be weaker, and you may feel you are chronically ill, instead of simply having had a "bout with cancer." You might, but hopefully you won't, develop a pervasive sense of uncertainty and feel helpless, with no sense of control. You may be angry that despite complying with treatment, you got sick again.

If fear of, or actual, recurrence is creating undue stress in your life, seek counseling or join a self-help group that addresses the matter supportively.

Problems of Caregivers

Throughout this book we have addressed the patient. Those who care about the patient will undoubtedly have learned much from it about diagnosis, treatments, and the problems facing the patient as he lives through cancer.

Those who care for and about the patient also need support. It is not easy to give emotional sustenance, to remain steadfast despite mood or behavioral changes, and to render physical care to a patient. Cancer gives a new dimension to the vow "for better or worse," and many spouses are as overwhelmed as the patient.

Often, family members have an even more difficult time than the patient in coping with the diagnosis and treatment plan. They may have conflicting feelings of love, fear, sorrow, pity, guilt, anger, and resentment. Any one or a combination of these emotions can cause tension, even interfering with proper treatment.

Well-meaning and loving family members may sometimes feel so overwhelmed that they become overprotective—or they may pretend nothing is the matter. Some try to take over the patient's life, making him feel as if he no longer has any control over anything. In some instances, the family may retreat from usual relations with the patient, causing a sense of loneliness and isolation for everyone. Families, as well as the patient, can benefit from recognition and discussion of these feelings; individual or group counseling is sometimes the best way to identify these problems and help you get a handle on them.

The cancer patient usually welcomes the support of others. If you listen and watch carefully, the patient will give clues to the kind of support he seeks. Whether you become a good listener, run errands, or assume some of his everyday chores—such as taking children or an elderly mother to the dentist—or just drop in with some neighborhood gossip, you can become an integral part of his support network.

Patients say they find it helpful when:

- you listen but don't tell them how they *should* feel.
- you don't give false or unknowing reassurance, which makes them feel as if you are discounting or are unaware of their fears.
- you tell them about *other* patients you know who have done well.
- you show them you understand that who they *are* is not related to what they *do*. Your former tennis or bridge partner needs to know he is still important to you even if he can't play.
- you ask for the patient's advice on matters about which they are knowledgeable.
- you find small but significant ways to help them—transportation to the doctor, errands, chores, etc.
- you sometimes just sit quietly.

More than ever, the crisis of cancer can give you, the friend or family member, an opportunity to express your feelings, and to let the patient know he is still an important person in your life.

Those With No Family or Close Friends

Such situations do exist. Perhaps you are living in a new location, far from old friends and family. Or you may be someone who has never formed close relationships, getting much of your emotional satisfaction from work. If you are unable to work, you may be removed from that support system.

Cancer is hard on anyone, perhaps hardest on those with no one to share the burden. Diminished energy may make it difficult to make new friends at this time. But it is not a hopeless endeavor.

Community and religious organizations, such as lodge, church, and temple groups, often welcome new members, even those who are unable to become actively involved. You may be able to make new friends among those you meet informally at the clinic or doctor's office or in a cancer support group. If you feel well enough, become a volunteer in some organization that interests you. Even sedentary work like stuffing envelopes can help fill your time and give you a sense of purpose as well as open new avenues of friendship.

Most communities have some sort of clearinghouse for volunteers. Call them. If you are homebound, many local agencies have a friendly visitor program, which can help ease your sense of isolation. A social worker at the hospital where your doctor is associated may have specific suggestions on how you can help others, and on how to meet new people.

Relaxation Techniques

Relaxation techniques can help relieve stress. Everyone has developed their own ways of relaxing: For some, it is jogging; for others, sitting back in a recliner chair and doing a crossword puzzle. Many of the techniques that you used in the past will still be effective for you, but others will no longer work, because they are too strenuous or require more concentration than you can presently muster. Or perhaps you never had any need for special relaxation techniques and will want to invent some.

This may be a time to learn some of the relaxation techniques that have been developed by experts in recent years, as discussed in Chapter 13. Some relaxation tapes may be available on loan from your local library or can be purchased, and some excellent books describe these techniques in detail. See Appendix VII.

Many psychologists, social workers, nurses, and other health professionals use relaxation methods as part of their treatment, and your doctor, nurse, or social worker may be able to recommend someone who can teach them to you. Other patients find that meditation or yoga is helpful.

Guided imagery, during which you visualize your cancer regressing and your healthy cells growing stronger, can also be psychologically beneficial; this technique is often taught along with relaxation methods. As I emphasized earlier, you should not confuse these techniques with a treatment for cancer. You should also know that imagery has not been proved to be statistically significant in helping treatment be more effective.

There are suggestions, but scanty evidence, that an optimistic attitude is helpful in the fight against cancer. However, if you feel more content and relaxed during the period in which you are receiving treatment, the quality of your life will certainly be improved. And that *is* very important.

Individual Counseling

As I've pointed out, many people manage to take their diagnosis in stride and learn to cope well, even though they have bad days from time to time. Such patients do not need counseling on a regular basis, but they often find it useful for sorting out feelings and concerns.

Other patients, and some family members, show such severe emotional reactions that counseling becomes essential. Often these reactions are related to underlying problems that have never been addressed. This may be the opportunity to discuss such problems and to resolve them.

Anxiety or depression that accompanies the side effects of chemotherapy and/or the diagnosis of cancer may be so severe that it cannot be alleviated by counseling alone. Your oncologist may recommend (or you can ask him to suggest) a consultation with a psychiatrist regarding medication and possible psychotherapy. In some instances, the oncologist himself may prescribe tranquilizers or antidepressants to relieve your anxiety or depression. Once you are more relaxed or calm, you may be more responsive to counseling. This combination—medication and the opportunity to discuss fears and concerns in a warm, accepting, professional relationship—can often be effective in helping you achieve a more positive outlook and return to normal everyday life.

Most patients will not need medication to help their anxiety or depression, but during counseling sessions they and family members can learn new ways to relate to each other, and to others, and to resolve old problems that have resurfaced during the illness.

Your doctor may be able to recommend a counselor to you who specializes in working with cancer patients, or you can telephone the social work department of the nearest major teaching hospital to ask for a referral. Those who counsel cancer patients are usually psychologists, social workers, nurses, or psychiatrists.

Group Counseling

Many cancer patients prefer group counseling to individual counseling. They hesitate to share these feelings with their doctor, family, or friends, for fear that those they need and care most about them will become irritated or angry. In a group of sympathetic strangers, however, they can share these feelings, or just listen to others talk about theirs. This can reduce stress on patients—as well as on family members, who frequently feel helpless because they cannot fully understand what their loved ones are experiencing.

Some groups are for patients only; others combine patients and those who figure significantly in their life. And there are groups only for spouses, family members or close friends, offering support and providing them with guidance to help the patient cope with his illness.

What happens in a good counseling group for cancer patients or their families? The pattern is the same for any group composed of people with a common problem: a sense of belonging and trust develops, transcending age, gender, education, and social status. A group does not exist for the purpose of offering false assurance but for expressing real feelings—for each person to gain and give to others strength and understanding during times of stress, and to rejoice in another's good news.

Group members will often displace their feelings and attitudes about people in their personal lives onto other members of the group. Guilt plays an important role in the patient's and family member's feelings, and in a group it can be discussed freely. The patient typically feels:

- What did I do to cause my disease?
- I'm complicating life for my family.
- I'm jealous and angry because others are healthy and I'm not.

Family members typically feel:

- What did I do to cause his disease?
- I feel sorry for him, but I resent all the new responsibilities I have because of his illness.
- I'm scared of what will happen to me if something happens to him.

Exploration and clarification of these and many other feelings in the safe, receptive atmosphere of the group diminishes anxiety and enables members to learn new and more effective ways of behaving, to develop greater sensitivity to others, and to become more realistic about their own feelings.

Groups serve another important function: This may be the only time a cancer patient can give, rather than receive, help.

But some patients do not want to be in groups. They would rather not be reminded that others are going through the same experience. If you don't feel a group is "right" for you, don't be coerced into joining one. Trust your own judgment. Others feel they would like a "kindred spirit," but still shy away from groups, so they form a relationship, either in person or by telephone, with another patient or two, and this gives them the kind of understanding and support they need.

If you or your family members or friends feel that you or they would benefit from group counseling, ask your doctor or the social work department of your local hospital if they know of any groups you can join.

Self-Help Groups

Self-help groups are generally composed of people in similar situations who can empathize with each other, share successes and failures, and provide emotional support and practical information. Sometimes these groups are started by social workers, nurses, or psychologists, but the responsibility for ongoing activities and continued meetings rests with the members.

Many hospitals, Y's, and other community agencies sponsor such groups. Across the country, over fifteen million people belong to more than half a million self-help groups of various kinds. In many cities, there is a "self-help clearinghouse," which can provide information on these groups. Your doctor, nurse, or the social work department at the hospital may have information on a group that meets your needs.

Some of these groups combine cancer patients, families, and friends all meeting together. Others are more clearly differentiated. Some patient groups are limited to those with specific types of cancers or undergoing particular procedures. Many groups concentrate on issues facing postmastectomy patients. Ostomy and laryngectomy groups, usually sponsored by the American Cancer Society, are essentially self-help groups. Appendix VI gives further information on some of these groups and programs.

If you feel that you prefer a self-help group to individual or group counseling, or would like to join one in addition to counseling, you should be able to find one in your area. You may even wish to begin one yourself; a social worker or other professional can offer you advice and training. Your local library or religious institution may be willing to help you publicize it and give you space in which to hold meetings.

Completion of treatment. Throughout the treatment period most patients eagerly await the day their oncologist tells them, "No more chemotherapy." But when the time finally arrives, many patients begin to panic. Suddenly "on their own," they fear that their cancer will return without the constant monitoring and treatment they have been receiving. Old conflicts and problems that had been put on the back burner may move up front as cancer treatment is no longer the focal point of the family's lives. Some patients, particularly those who had surgery prior to treatment, suddenly begin to mourn a lost body part or function. Therapists who work with cancer patients say that the end of treatment is a crisis for many patients, and that counseling can be very helpful at this time.

The emotional impact of cancer can be great. For the most part, people cope with cancer in much the same way they have coped with other crises in the past. Family and friends can be a big help. Severe depression or anxiety can be treated; counseling is available for anyone who feels they need it. Although each patient and family unit is unique, knowing that others are going through similar experiences can be helpful.

No one has to "go it alone." Seek help, and live your life as fully as you can.

Chapter 17

What Shall We Tell the Children?

You may be comfortable speaking openly of your disease and treatment with other adults but hesitate to tell your children or grandchildren for fear of upsetting them.

Child-development experts usually agree that children can be told most things if they are told about it in a way they can understand, and one that is sensitive to any fears they have. Even a fairly young child can be told, "Daddy has a tumor on his back and the doctor is going to take it off. A tumor is a growth that shouldn't be there, so that's why the doctor is removing it. Then another doctor is going to give him some very strong medicine that goes right into his body and helps to keep the tumor from growing back."

Later, the child might notice the effects of treatment. You could say, "Yes, the medicine is so strong that it sometimes makes him very sick. Daddy has a good doctor who cares very much about keeping him well, and that's why he needs to take the medicine."

In this way, you are reassuring your child that everyone is doing their best, and that many people care about Daddy.

But don't make promises you can't keep. No child should be promised that both parents will still be around to pack him off to college, but you *can* promise that someone will always be there to take care of him, to take him to school, go shopping, fix favorite foods, and to read him a bedtime story.

It would be wise to advise the child's teacher and school principal when a parent or very close grandparent is undergoing treatment. They may be able to help the youngster through some difficult times, and they will remain alert to any changes in study habits or behavior.

Children's fears of parental illness often focus on "What will become of me?" rather than "Poor Mommy [or Daddy]." This is a normal reaction for both children and adolescents, and is important to keep in mind. They may be upset when a grandparent is ill for some of the same reasons. They may feel that if Grandmother is sick, Mother can also get sick, thus abandoning them. An ill grandparent can also take time and attention away from a child, upsetting the security of his everyday world.

Children sometimes feel guilty, believing that something they did or thought is responsible for causing a parent or grandparent to become ill. Children feel that they can make all kinds of bad things happen, and you should look for opportunities to reassure them that they are in no way responsible for this illness.

Thus, it is not a good idea to tell a child that if he is very good, it will help a parent get better. Then, when a parent isn't feeling well, the child may feel he wasn't "good enough." But you *can* tell a child that his crayon drawings helped cheer up your room; that his hugs and kisses made you feel better, and that the gelatin he made was the best thing you ate all week.

Generally speaking, your instincts about discussing cancer and treatment with your children will lead you to handling it well. You will recognize your children's feelings, fears, and fantasies, and will discuss them in a serious but matter-of-fact manner. You may have to remind yourself not to ask adolescents to assume too much responsibility for younger children in the home or for housekeeping chores, thus robbing them of their youth and risking rebellion later.

Many parents would rather not speak with children about cancer, because they may also wish to protect children from such unpleasantness. But children do know; sometimes they overhear conversations or pick up clues from your behavior. This can cause more worry than if you explain things to them.

Children often worry that cancer is catching, and it is important that you tell them it isn't. They may also have the idea that everyone who develops cancer dies; they may have heard about some celebrity who died of cancer, or even know someone who died of it. It's important that they know that many people live a long time with cancer and that it can often be cured. Some parents promise to tell their children that they will let them know if things aren't going well; this way, children won't have to keep guessing.

Some children feel very excluded when a parent is ill. Grandma, who always used to have time for the children, may now appear to be more concerned and involved with the parent who is getting treatment than with the children. This can make a child very jealous and angry.

In addition to feelings of exclusion, a child may feel "different" because he has a parent with cancer. He needs to be reassured that he is still the same person he was before his parent became ill. Many children feel much more a part of things if they can speak with the parent's oncologist. An alternative plan might be to ask the doctor to speak with your pediatrician, who in turn can explain the medical situation to the child. Social workers and nurses can also do this. Allowing children to get "first-hand" information gives them a sense of participation and inclusion. Here are some guidelines to remember, regarding children of all ages:

Be sure that someone tells them you have cancer, because:

- They are bound to learn about it anyway.
- They may be more worried than necessary and have all sorts of fantasies about what will happen to *you* and to *them*.
- They won't think you are protecting them if you withold information; they will just feel excluded and may even think their feelings don't matter to you.
- If you have to keep a secret, you will always be "on guard," and this may make you retreat from close interaction.

The people best suited to discuss this problem with the children are:

- you, if you feel you can discuss it calmly. A few tears are O.K., but if you think you will sound angry or depressed, or are unable to cope with the discussion, let someone else talk to them.
- another adult who knows the children well: a relative, their best friend's parent, or another trusted adult, such as a school guidance counselor or teacher. Try to be present or available right after the conversation.
- your doctor or the child's doctor.

The best time to tell the children is:

- as soon as anyone else knows.

The best way to tell children is:

- in person—not on the phone.
- with honesty, but as optimistically as possible.
- when you have plenty of time to answer their questions. Leave plenty of time for questions, and if they don't have any, ask them, "How do you feel about what I have told you?" Let them know that if they have questions later, they can ask you, and if they are old enough, you can suggest they write their questions down if you aren't available when they think about them. But don't force them to talk about it.
- in a manner appropriate to their age. The youngest children can be told that you have a sickness and will get treatment; sometimes

the treatment may make you sick. There will always be someone to take care of them, even if the parent isn't well (or is in the hospital). Older children need that same reassurance but may prefer more specific information, and may want to read a bit about cancer.

Some tips for day-to-day living:

- Try to keep the family's routine as stable as possible, even if it means reassigning roles or asking others for help.
- Aim for consistency in dealing with small children. If you need to make child-care arrangements, try not to keep changing people.
- It won't hurt the kids not to eat home-cooked, balanced meals every single day. Fast-food restaurants can be a boon to a parent who is trying to juggle hospital visits or who isn't up to cooking.
- Let the neighbors help out by inviting the kids over. You can reciprocate when you feel better, or make up for it with little gifts.
- Relax some of the children's rules, but don't become too permissive. They may think no one cares about them anymore.

Most children would rather *not*:

- know about things that may not actually happen. Thus, don't discuss possible biopsy reports until they are completed, or the need for surgery if it has not yet been determined.
- be promised something if you can't be certain the promise will be kept. Don't say, "We'll all go to Disneyland next summer," if it may turn out that you can't go.
- be lied to *ever*. If you don't know something, admit it.
- be given more responsibility than they think they can handle, even if *you* feel they can.
- hear too much about money problems, although it is reasonable to let them know that they can't have everything they want.
- feel different from other kids. Even a college freshman can be embarrassed to see a parent with a cane or in a wheelchair on visiting day. Don't think they will always be self-centered and uncaring—it's just a "stage."
- be made to feel guilty for not doing enough or not seeming to care enough. They do care but often have strange ways of showing it.
- be left out of things.
- be forced to visit a sick parent or grandparent in the hospital, or stay at home with them when they want to go somewhere else. Often they are not selfish, just trying to protect themselves from a painful situation.

Some children and adolescents may become troubled by the situation, despite all your honesty and reassurances. Some of the signs you should be alert to are:

- School phobias (continual reluctance or refusal to go to school).
- Attention-seeking behavior (aggressiveness, constant arguments, defiance, rule-breaking, etc.).
- Sleep and eating disturbances (too much or too little).
- "Too-good" behavior.
- Excessive quietness (indicating sadness, fear, or depression).
- Regressive (babyish) behavior.
- Overidentification with the ill parent, resulting in physical symptoms that have no medical basis.
- Bed-wetting (if it had already stopped).

If you notice any of the above signs, it would be wise to consult with a mental-health professional who is experienced in dealing with children's needs, fears, and anxieties. This person might be a school nurse, school guidance counselor, child psychologist, psychiatrist, or social worker. Your pediatrician or a medical social worker at the hospital where your oncologist is associated should be able to recommend a good counselor who can help you find out if there really is a problem, and then guide your family to "getting it all together again."

Tell yourself every day, and be ready to tell it to your kids, too:

- I didn't make myself sick.
- My spouse didn't make me sick.
- My children didn't make me sick.
- Cancer made me sick.

Some children truly suffer when a parent is ill, and if the parent does not recover, the loss may have a profound effect. But many children and adolescents who have a trying time when a parent has cancer come through the experience—with time, and sometimes counseling—more empathetic human beings with a greater appreciation for the important things in life.

Afterword

Some cancers—such as Hodgkin's disease, lymphatic leukemia, lymphomas, choriocarcinoma, testicular tumors, certain sarcomas, and some carcinomas—are often curable nowadays. Almost half of all cancer patients are alive five years after diagnosis. (This statistic does not include those with nonmelanoma skin cancer or carcinoma in situ, or those who have died as a result of accident or unrelated disease.) More than one third of all people who develop cancer today can be considered cured. The rate would be even higher if diagnosis and treatment were made and started earlier. A number of cancers once thought to be incurable can be so well controlled that many patients are surviving for several years after treatment.

Each year we hear about more breakthroughs in cancer treatment, but all of us who care for or about cancer patients are painfully aware that some people simply do not have long-term response to treatment.

But to the patient and his family, even "long-term" is never long enough. Patients and families alike, we all bargain for that extra time, even as we attempt to cram a lifetime of living into the days following the diagnosis.

As I began work on this book, my brother-in-law was diagnosed with carcinoma of the lung. Now, as I complete these pages, it is more than a year since he began chemotherapy. In between visits to the doctor's office and hospitalizations for treatment with cis-platinum, he has continued to work, play golf, and, to his particular pleasure, attend Giants football games. Together our families have celebrated birthdays, holidays, wedding anniversaries, a law-school graduation, and then, just as the one-year anniversary of his diagnosis came along, the joy to which every father looks forward. He walked his youngest daughter down the aisle, stood on the receiving line, and danced with the bride, her sister, his wife, and innumerable guests. It has been a rough year, and we all know it. But it has also been a year full of love, and we all know that, too.

I thought often of my mother as I wrote this book. At sixty she was diagnosed with cancer of the breast, and following her surgery she had radiation therapy. She remained well for twelve years, during which time she watched five grandchildren grow from youngsters to young adults. She attended several high-school and college graduations, toasted a granddaughter at her wedding, and with my father, celebrated their fiftieth anniversary and his eightieth birthday. And when her cancer recurred, she underwent chemotherapy with her usual indomitable spirit. During her last months we talked openly, and although I miss her still, I am grateful for those fourteen years that the best state-of-the-art treatment could offer her in 1964, and again in 1976.

And so I am keenly aware that no handbook for cancer patients would be complete without a discussion of the problems that arise when treatment is no longer effective.

In the chapter about the team approach, I discussed visiting nurses and home care. Throughout the country, hospitals and community programs have joined together to try to help cancer patients and their families cope with the care of the very ill patient.

Many of these programs are called home oncology medical extension programs, or hospices. They are specialized health-care programs that emphasize the management of pain and other symptoms associated with advanced or terminal illness. Quality of life is the primary concern of these programs, and while most support is palliative, it is not restricted to that type of care; when treatment is indicated, it is offered. An interdisciplinary team is available, usually consisting of a medical oncologist, a psychiatrist, an oncology nurse, a social worker, and a medical technologist. A nutritionist, physical therapist, pharmacist, clergy and volunteers, are often available as well. In cooperation with the local visiting-nurse service, regular home nursing and homemaking may also be provided.

Such services allow patients to remain at home, and let families participate in their care. Many, but not all, patients and their families find this preferable to lengthy hospitalization.

The original concept of *hospice*, as conceived by Dr. Cicely Saunders in England in 1967 at St. Christopher's Hospice, was a place separate from any hospital, for the dying and their families to receive support and help rather than continued treatment if it was no longer of any value to the patient.

In the United States today, a hospice may be an actual independent institution, but many are located within a hospital or skilled nursing facility, and still more take the form of home-care programs associated with a hospital. When hospitalization is needed, the patient can be transferred there, and then returned home again, if that is the patient and family's choice.

To learn more about hospice care, and to get the names of hospices in your area, contact the National Hospice Organization (see Appendix VI).

Cancer touches most of our lives in some way. In the struggle against it, you and your family's understanding of the disease and treatment can help you to obtain the best treatment known today, and to achieve a high quality of life. I hope that this book has proved useful, and that you are one of the millions of people now living a normal life despite cancer.

January 1986
New York City

Appendixes

Appendix I

Questions to Ask Your Physician

Please remember that every patient and his response to the illness and treatment is different, so your doctor may not be able to answer all these questions precisely. And some may simply not be relevant for you.

What type of cancer do I have, and can you tell me the exact cell type and stage at the time of diagnosis?

Has there been any spread beyond where it began that you *know* about? That you suspect? That often occurs, even if diagnostic tests do not reveal it?

If there is no evidence of spread, how will I be watched to be sure it *doesn't* spread?

What are the risks of the surgical procedure you are recommending?

What are the risks of not having the surgery [or other recommended treatment]?

How will my everyday functioning be affected by this treatment?

If I need radiotherapy, what type will I get? Internal? External?

Will I need to be hospitalized for radiotherapy? If so, for how long?

If I need chemotherapy, will I get it in the hospital or in an office or clinic?

How long will I need to be treated?

How often and for how long will I need to return for checkups relating to this cancer?

Will you be scheduling regular tests? What tests?

What will those tests tell us?

What are the particular signs of recurrence to which I should be alert?

In addition to these questions, please consult Section Two, which describes the various treatments for different cancers.

Appendix II

When to Call Your Physician

If you are undergoing (or have undergone) treatment for cancer and notice any of these symptoms, telephone your doctor's office. Do *not* wait until your next visit.

- Temperature over 100° F., taken orally (buy a thermometer *before* you need it).
- Chills or tremors.
- Bleeding.
- Severe or persistent pain, anywhere.
- Severe or persistent headache.
- Shortness of breath.
- Inability or difficulty in "catching" your breath.
- Sudden weight gain or loss.
- Skin rashes or mouth sores.
- Infections, boils, or abscesses.
- Severe constipation or diarrhea.
- Urinary retention (inability or severe difficulty in urinating).
- Urinary incontinence (inability to hold back urine).
- Blood in urine or stool.
- Severe and persistent vomiting, nausea, diarrhea, or heartburn.
- Severe pain at injection site.
- Exposure to any contagious disease, especially chicken pox, shingles, or any variety of herpes.
- Swelling of hands, feet, or eyelids.
- Bruising or several black-and-blue marks.
- Persistent cough or hoarseness.
- Persistent dizziness or blurred vision.
- Difficulty in walking.
- Changes in menstrual cycle or flow.

None of these symptoms necessarily means that you are experiencing a toxic reaction to treatment or a recurrence of the cancer, but they should be evaluated by your oncologist.

Appendix III
Drugs That Can Interfere with a Treatment Plan

Do not take any of the following prescription or nonprescription drugs without first consulting your oncologist.

- Alka-Seltzer.
- Antibiotics.
- Anticoagulants (or any medication for blood disorders).
- Anticonvulsant (antiseizure) pills, such as Dilantin.
- Antidepressants.
- Antidiarrhea medication.
- Antihistamines.
- Barbiturates, such as Seconal or Nembutal.
- Blood-pressure pills.
- Cough medicines.
- Diuretics.
- Insulin, or any oral medication for diabetes.
- Laxatives.
- Nose sprays.
- Pain medication, including aspirin, Bufferin, Tylenol, Anacin, iboprufin.
- Sleeping pills.
- Tranquilizers.
- Vitamins.

Do not take any flu shots or vaccines, either, without first consulting your oncologist.

Appendix IV

Patient's Personal Records

You can take an active role in your own care by keeping careful records of your tests and treatments. In addition, you should keep in a convenient place the names and telephone numbers of those health-care professionals who are part of your team. You will need a loose-leaf notebook and a supply of blank pages to add as necessary.

Page One: *Important names and telephone numbers*
Medical oncologist, surgeon, radiotherapist, family doctor, dentist, local emergency service, nurse at clinic or doctor's office, visiting nurse, social worker, physical and/or occupational therapist, nutritionist/dietician, local pharmacy, nearest twenty-four-hour pharmacy, hospital pharmacy, homemaker agency, medical-equipment supplier, ambulance company, nurse's aid, nursing agency, Homemaker Agency, neighbors.
Photocopy the above and post it near your telephone. Give copies to a close friend, neighbor, or relative.

Page Two: *Diagnostic tests*
List dates, names of tests, and office or hospital where each test was performed, results, and any future schedule of surgical biopsies, X rays, scans, and other tests.

Page Three: *Hospitalizations*
List dates of admission and discharge, name of hospital, reason for admission, name of physician, and, if possible, your chart or unit number.

Page Four: *Chemotherapy*
List names of all drugs, whether given by injections or taken orally, and dates. If you're on a specific schedule, list dates you are supposed to take the medications.

250

Page Five: *Other drugs*
> List any drugs—such as aspirin, pain medication, anti-inflammatory drugs, vitamins—frequency taken, and by whom it was suggested or prescribed.

Page Six: *Radiation*
> List any radiation you have had. For external radiation, list all dates, type of machine, location on body, number of rads, and hospital or office in which it was administered. For internal radiation, list date of implant, hospital or office where it was made, type of implant, location in body of the implant, and if removed, date of removal.

Page Seven: *Things to tell your physician*
> This page is valuable for everyone, but especially so for someone who lives alone. You may wish to photocopy this page, sign it, and give it to your physician to place in your chart and also give a copy to someone else. List (1) legal next of kin, relationship; (2) a person whom you might prefer to identify as "my next of kin," although he/she is not legally so; (3) any person/people you feel may best be able to give you emotional support; (4) the person/people with whom the physician has permission to discuss your medical condition at any time (include doctors, relatives, and/or friends, attorney/s, or someone else). If you do not want your doctor to discuss your medical condition with anyone (except physicians, nurses, therapists, social workers, and other health-care professionals) *without* your permission (unless you become physically or mentally incompetent), make this statement, sign and date it.
> *Be sure to give full addresses and telephone numbers for anyone you have listed here.*

Appendix V

Drugs Used in Cancer Chemotherapy

Since reactions to drugs vary greatly among individuals, some side effects may occur that are not listed here. Likewise, many of the side effects listed below may not be experienced by all patients or may be so mild that they are not noticed. Since this list serves only as a guideline, report to your physician if these or *any* unexpected symptoms develop. Unusual and rare side effects are not included in this list.

Names (Brand Names indicated by ®)	Type of Drug (chemical categories) (Hormone Section starts on Pg. 256)	Type of Cancer (examples of cancer for which drug is used)	Possible Side Effects
Asparaginase L'Asparaginase (Elspar®)	anti–amino acid	acute lymphoblastic leukemia	skin, allergic and pulmonary reactions, nausea, vomiting, pancreatic bleeding, lowered blood counts, lethargy and depression
Bleomycin (Blenoxane®)	antitumor antibiotic	squamous-cell carcinomas; head and neck, cervix, skin, testicular, Hodgkin's and Non-Hodgkin's lymphomas, lung	pulmonary, skin rash and flushing, nail changes, hair loss, mouth sores, fever, chills, vomiting, weight loss, loss of appetite, allergic reactions
Busulfan (Myleran®)	alkylating agent	chronic myelogenous leukemias	lowered blood counts, tiredness, skin and pulmonary reactions, enlarged male breasts, amenorrhea, nausea, weight loss
Carmustine BCNU (BiCNU®)	alkylating agent (nitrosourea)	brain, melanoma, colon, stomach, pancreas, lung, Hodgkin's and Non-Hodgkin's lymphomas, liver, multiple myeloma	nausea, vomiting, lowered blood counts, liver or lung pain, local venous pain on administration

Names (Brand Names indicated by ®)	Type of Drug (chemical categories) (Hormone Section starts on Pg. tk)	Type of Cancer (examples of cancer for which drug is used)	Possible Side Effects
Chlorambucil (Leukeran®)	alkylating agent	breast, chronic lymphocytic leukemia, ovarian, Hodgkin's and Non-Hodgkin's lymphomas	nausea, lowered blood counts
Cisplatin Cisplatinum Platinum Compound (Platinol®)	alkylating agent	ovarian, testicular, lung, head and neck, bladder, prostate, osteogenic sarcoma, cervix	severe nausea, vomiting, ringing in ears, decreased hearing, dulling or loss of sensation in arms and legs, joint pain, lowered blood counts, kidney damage
Cyclophosphamide (Cytoxan®, Neosar®)	alkylating agent	lymphomas, leukemias, breast, lung, ovary, myeloma, cervix, neuroblastoma, sarcomas	bladder infection, hair loss, lowered blood counts, loss of appetite, nausea or vomiting, nail changes, problems with fluid balance
Cytarabine ARA C Cytosine Arabinoside (Cytosar-U®)	antimetabolite	myelocytic and lymphocytic leukemias, Hodgkin's and Non-Hodgkin's lymphomas	lowered blood counts, nausea, vomiting
Dacarbazine DTIC Imidazole Carboxamide (DTIC-Dome®)	atypical alkylating agent	melanoma, Hodgkin's disease, sarcomas	lowered blood counts, loss of appetite, nausea, vomiting, fever and weakness, venous irritation on administration
Dactinomycin Actinomycin D (Cosmegen®)	antitumor antibiotic	Wilms' tumor, rhabdomyosarcoma, testicular, uterine, choriocarcinoma, sarcomas	nausea, vomiting, lowered blood counts, diarrhea, mouth sores, hair loss, skin eruptions, venous irritation on administration, acne
Daunorubicin Daunomycin Rubidomycin (Cerubidine®)	antimetabolite	acute lymphocytic and nonlymphocytic leukemias	cardiac, lowered blood counts, hair loss, nausea, vomiting, red urine, fever, venous irritation on administration
Doxorubicin (Adriamycin®)	antitumor antibiotic	granulocytic and lymphocytic leukemias, Non-Hodgkin's and Hodgkin's lym-	cardiac, lowered blood counts, nausea, vomiting, mouth sores, hair loss, red urine

Names (Brand Names indicated by ®)	Type of Drug (chemical categories) (Hormone Section starts on Pg. tk)	Type of Cancer (examples of cancer for which drug is used)	Possible Side Effects
		phomas, stomach, breast, lung, ovarian, liver, sarcoma, bladder, endometrial, neuroblastoma, prostate, head and neck, testicular, thyroid, Wilms' tumor	
Estramustine (Emcyt®)	nitrogen mustard plus Estradiol	prostate	nausea, vomiting, diarrhea, enlargement of male breast
Etoposide VP 16 (VePesid®)	mitotic inhibitor (podophyllotoxin)	testicular, lung, lymphomas, leukemias	constipation, hair loss, nerve disorders, low blood counts, nausea, vomiting
Floxuridine (FUDR®)	antimetabolite	liver	nausea, vomiting, diarrhea, mouth sores, flushing, lowered blood counts, loss of appetite
Flourouracil 5-Fluorouracil 5-FU (Fluorouracil®, (Adrucil®, Efudex®	antimetabolite	colon, rectum, breast, stomach, pancreas, bladder, liver, ovarian, cervix (topical use for basal-cell and squamous-cell skin cancers)	nausea, vomiting, diarrhea, mouth sores, lowered blood counts, nail changes, hair loss
Hydroxyurea (Hydrea®)	antimetabolite	chronic myelogeneous leukemia, head and neck, kidney, melanoma, prostate	lowered blood counts, nausea, vomiting, diarrhea, constipation, mouth sores, rash
Lomustine CCNU (CeeNU®)	alkylating agent (nitrosourea)	brain, melanoma, colon, lung, Hodgkin's disease	nausea, vomiting, loss of appetite, lowered blood counts, hair loss
Mechlorethamine (Mustargen®)	alkylating agent	Hodgkin's disease, lymphomas, lung	nausea, vomiting, hair loss, lowered blood counts, metallic taste
Melphalan L'PAM L'phenylalanine mustard L'sarcolysin (Alkeran®)	alkylating agent	multiple myeloma, ovarian, breast, testicular, melanoma	lowered blood counts, nausea, vomiting, diarrhea, mouth sores, skin eruption

254

Names (Brand Names indicated by ®)	Type of Drug (chemical categories) (Hormone Section starts on Pg. tk)	Type of Cancer (examples of cancer for which drug is used)	Possible Side Effects
Mercaptopurine 6-Mercaptopurine (Purinethol®)	antimetabolite (purine analogue)	acute or chronic myelogenous and acute lymphatic leukemias	nausea, vomiting, loss of appetite, lowered blood counts, liver
Methotrexate MTX Amethopterin (Methotrexate® Mexate®, Folex®)	antimetabolite	breast, cervix, head and neck, leukemias, lymphomas, choriocarcinoma, lung, medulloblastoma, micosis fungoides, ostoegenic and rhabdomyosarcomas	mouth sores, nausea, vomiting, diarrhea, lowered blood counts, liver, kidney, pulmonary
Mitomycin Mitomycin C (Mutamycin®)	antitumor antibiotic	gastric, pancreas, colon, breast, lung	lowered blood counts, nausea, vomiting, kidney
Mitotane o,p'-DDD (Lysodren®)	anti-adrenal gland	adrenal	nausea, vomiting, loss of appetite, diarrhea, confusion, vision changes, skin rash
Plicamycin (Mithracin®)	antitumor antibiotic	testicular	lowered blood counts, nausea, vomiting, mouth sores, loss of appetite, liver, kidney, headache, lethargy, skin rash
Procarbazine (Matulane®)	miscellaneous	Hodgkin's disease, lymphomas, lung, brain	lowered blood counts, nausea, vomiting, muscle or joint pain, lethargy, depression, severe reaction with alcohol
Streptozocin (Zanosar®)	antitumor antibiotic (nitrosourea)	islet cell and other pancreatic, Hodgkin's disease, carcinoid tumors	nausea, vomiting, lowered blood counts, low blood sugar leading to weakness and headaches, kidney damage
Thioguanine 6-Thioguanine	antimetabolite (purine analogue)	acute nonlymphocytic and lymphocytic leukemias	lowered blood counts
Thio-TEPA (Thiotepa®)	alkylating agent	breast, ovarian, bladder, Hodgkin's disease	lowered blood counts, loss of appetite
Vinblastine (Velban®)	mitotic inhibitor (vinca alkaloid)	Hodgkin's and Non-Hodgkin's lymphomas, tes-	lowered blood counts, constipation, hair loss, abdominal pain,

Names (Brand Names indicated by ®)	Type of Drug (chemical categories) (Hormone Section starts on Pg. tk)	Type of Cancer (examples of can- cer for which drug is used)	Possible Side Effects
		ticular, breast, choriocarcinoma	nerve disorders, nau- sea, vomiting, mouth sores
Vincristine (Oncovin®)	mitotic inhibitor (vinca alkaloid)	leukemias, lym- phomas, Hodg- kin's disease, breast, sarcomas, neuroblastoma, Wilms' tumor	hair loss, constipa- tion, nerve disorders, jaw pain, abdominal pain

New drugs are constantly being developed that are effective against specific types of cancer. Usage of the individual agents, singly and in combination, are constantly being evaluated. Changes will occur even as you read this book.

HORMONES SECTION

Group	Types of Cancer	Side Effects
Adrenocorticoids		
Betamethasone (Celestone) Dexamethasone (Decadron) Hydrocortisone (Solu-Cortef) Prednisolone Prednisone	lymphomas, Hodg- kin's disease, acute leukemias, breast, myeloma, chronic lymphocytic leuke- mia	increased appetite and sense of well being, abnormal hair growth, fluid retention, increased risk of infection, mood swings, acnelike rash, weight gain, ulcers, abnor- mal fat accumulation, muscle weakness, thinning of skin, elevated blood sugar (diabetes)
Androgens		
Fluoxymesterone (Halotestin) Methyltestosterone (Oreton) Nandrolone (Deca- Durabolin) Testolactone (Teslac) Testosterone	breast	fluid retention, nausea and vomiting, water retention, weight gain, changes in li- bido, disruption in men- struation, liver toxicity, elevated calcium, lowering of voice, hair growth
Antiestrogens		
Tamoxifen (Nolvadex)	breast	transient nausea and vomit- ing, hot flashes, light-head- edness, vaginal discharge, itching, headache
Estrogens		
Chlorotrianisene (Tace)	breast, prostate	nausea, vomiting, fluid re- tention, weight gain, swol-

256

Group	Types of Cancer	Side Effects
Diethylstilbestrol (DES) Estradiol (Estrace)		len tender breasts, headache, GI symptoms, disruption of menstruation, loss of calcium, uterine bleeding, libido, elevated
Progestogens		
Hydroxyprogesterone (Delalutin) Medroxyprogesterone (Depo-Provera) Megestrol (Megace)	kidney, breast, prostatic, endometrial	mild side effects including GI symptoms, decreased libido, breast enlargement or tenderness

INVESTIGATIONAL AGENTS

Amsacrine	Hexamethylmelamine	Mitoxantrone
Azacitidine	(HMM)	Semustine (Methyl-
Bisantrene	Ifosfamide (Ifex)	CCNU)
Carboplatin	Interferon	Tegafur (Ftorafur)
Cyproterone	Leuprolide	Teniposide (VM-26)
Deoxycoformycin	Mitobronitol	Vindesine (Eldisine)
Flutamide	Mitolactol	

The above drugs are presently undergoing clinical trials, which means that they are available to some patients. In order to be treated with "investigational" drugs, you must sign an "informed consent," meaning that you understand that the risks and/or benefits from these drugs are not yet fully known by your oncologist. Data will have been collected on some of these agents and they will be available as standard cancer treatment by your oncologist by the time you read this book.

(Prepared by Jaclyn Silverman)

Appendix VI
Reference Guide to Further Information

The National Cancer Institute supports cancer research throughout the country, and also conducts its own research. Especially useful and valuable to cancer patients and their families is NCI's information and referral service. This service is called the Cancer Information Service (CIS) of the National Cancer Institute. The toll-free phone numbers to reach them are:

In the continental United States (except the Washington, D.C., area): 1-800-4-CANCER
In Hawaii: 808-524-1234 (local in Oahu; from neighboring islands, call collect)
In Washington, D.C. (and suburbs in Maryland and Virginia): 202-636-5700.
In Alaska: 1-800-638-6070.

When you call the CIS number, you are connected with the regional office serving your area. They can give you accurate, personalized answers to your cancer-related questions, and can tell you about various community agencies and services available, and where you can find a medical library near your home. Upon request, they will give you the name of the closest Comprehensive Cancer Center and tell you where any experimental programs for your type of cancer are being conducted. If you wish, they will guide you in finding a private physician, and in some instances they can give you the names of specific physicians.

Spanish-speaking staff members are available to callers from the following areas (daytime hours only): California (213, 714, 619, 809, and 818), Florida, Georgia, Illinois, northern New Jersey, New York City, and Texas.

You can write to them for a list of written materials available on cancer in general, or on specific types of cancer, at the following address:

Office of Cancer Communications
National Cancer Institute (NCI)
National Institutes of Health
Building 31, Room 1018A
Bethesda, MD 20014

The American Cancer Society, in addition to funding research, sponsors several patient-support programs, such as Reach to Recovery (a patient-to-patient service for mastectomy patients), I Can Cope (an educational program for patients and families), CanSurmount (a patient-to-patient support service), and programs of the International Association of Laryngectomees and United Ostomy Associations. Many local ACS divisions and units can help with transportation (either with financial aid or through a program called Road to Recovery), and some offer care in the home.

Look in your local telephone directory for the nearest American Cancer Society division or unit. They can give you information about locally available services and provide you with various written materials. If you are unable to find the local division, contact the national office:

American Cancer Society (ACS)
National Headquarters
90 Park Avenue
New York, NY 10016
212-599-8200

The Canadian Cancer Society offers many of the same services as the American Cancer Society and maintains divisions in each of the provinces. Check the telephone directory service to locate the division nearest you, or call their national office:

The Canadian Cancer Society
130 Bloor Street West
Suite 1001
Toronto, Ontario
Canada M5S 2V7
416-961-7223

The United Cancer Council is a federation of voluntary cancer agencies whose primary emphasis is on patient services. Local member agencies throughout the country offer financial help, loan of equipment, cancer counseling, transportation, homemaking, and other services to cancer patients and their families. They also support research.

Many of their member agencies, such as Cancer Care, Inc., and Make Today Count, are listed below. A request by mail or phone to the United Cancer Council will put you in touch with a local agency. If no agency is in your area, the council will often offer help directly to you. Call or write:

United Cancer Council, Inc.
650 East Carmel Drive
Carmel, IN 46032
317-844-6627

The National Self-Help Clearinghouse has a list of local clearinghouses throughout the country that can refer you to self-help groups in your area. Send a self-addressed stamped envelope, with your request for the name of the clearinghouse nearest you, to:

National Self-Help Clearinghouse
Graduate School and University Center of the City University of
  New York
33 West 42nd Street
New York, NY 10036

Cancer Care, a division of the National Cancer Foundation, is a voluntary social-service agency that provides professional counseling and planning by social workers to cancer patients and their families. Direct services, which include financial assistance, are available to residents of New York, New Jersey, and Connecticut. Programs of professional consultation and education, social research, public affairs, and public education on a national and worldwide basis are also available. Write or call:

Cancer Care, Inc. of the National Cancer Foundation
1180 Avenue of the Americas
New York, NY 10020
212-221-3300
212-302-2400 (direct line for referrals to social work department)

CHUMS (Cancer Hopefuls United for Mutual Support) offers emotional support to cancer patients, families and friends, and fights for the rights of cancer patients, especially in the areas of employment and insurance. They also offer information through their newsletter. Send a self-addressed, stamped envelope for information.

CHUMS
3310 Rochambeau Avenue
New York, NY 10467
212-655-7566

The Leukemia Society of America provides financial assistance and agency referrals to patients with leukemia and related diseases, such as lymphoma, multiple myeloma, pre-leukemia, and Hodgkin's disease. For further information, write:

Leukemia Society of America, Inc.
733 Third Avenue
New York, NY 10017

Make Today Count is an all-volunteer self-help support group that brings together cancer patients, other seriously ill people, and concerned members of the community to help improve quality of life by indentifying problems and helping people cope with them. Founded by the late Orville Kelly in 1973, the organization has local chapters nationwide; their common goal is "living each day as fully and completely as possible." For the name of a chapter near you, call or write:

Make Today Count, Inc.
P.O. Box 222
Osage Beach, MO 65065
314-348-1619

The National HomeCaring Council provides information about selecting appropriate home care for the ill and disabled. Write to:

National HomeCaring Council, Inc.
235 Park Avenue South
New York, NY 10003

The National Hospice Organization publishes brochures and pamphlets on hospice care. They will also give you the names of hospices near you. Write or call:

National Hospice Organization
1901 North Fort Myer Drive
Suite 902
Arlington, VA 22209
703-243-5900

SIECUS (Sex Information and Education Council of the U.S.) will provide information on books, periodicals, and organizations relating to sexuality and illness. Send $1 and a stamped, self-addressed #10 envelope, requesting this list: *Sexuality and Disability: A Bibliography of Resources Available for Purchase.*

SIECUS
80 Fifth Avenue
New York, NY 10011

The United Ostomy Association provides supportive and informational services, and sponsors self-help groups for those who have had an ostomy. Trained volunteers from many local chapters meet with patients on a patient-to-patient basis, helping them to adjust to their ostomy. For a list of publications and for information about one of the nationwide ostomy groups in your area, write:

United Ostomy Association, Inc.
2001 West Beverly Boulevard
Los Angeles, CA 90057
213-413-5510

In Canada
Hamilton District Ostomy Association
5 Hamilton Avenue
Hamilton, Ontario L8V 2S3
416-389-8822

To find a medical oncologist

If your physician or the hospital nearest you cannot recommend an oncologist, you can call the county medical society and ask for a referral. They will probably give you three names. You can also look in the *Directory of Medical Specialists*, which lists all physicians who are American board-certified specialists. A new directory is issued every two years. Your branch library may have it; if not, the librarian can tell you where to find it. Following the section entitled "American Board of Internal Medicine," you will find the various subspecialties. Look for "Medical Oncology," and under that look for the community nearest you. (You can find the name of any specialist in this way.)

If you wish to check the credentials or affiliations of any board-certified physician, you can look up his name in the alphabetical index of the directory, which will then tell you on what page he is listed.

Most states have a medical directory of all state-licensed physicians, which is probably available in your local library. The American Medical Association (AMA) also publishes a directory of physicians in the United States. These books are good sources for information on physicians. Your local medical society may also be able to give you referrals.

You may also contact:

American Society of Clinical Oncologists
435 North Michigan Avenue
Chicago, IL 60611
312-644-0828

This association will give you the names of several oncologists (medical, surgical radiation, or pediatric) in your area. All are board-certified or board-eligible oncologists. You can also ask them if a specific physician you've met or been referred to is one of the society's members (who number more than five thousand).

To find a pain specialist

Call the Cancer Information Service toll-free number (listed at the beginning of this appendix) to find the name of the nearest university- or hospital-based pain clinic. If this clinic is too far from your home for you to be treated there, your physician can consult doctors there by phone, or they can recommend a pain specialist near you. Your county medical society may also be able to give you a referral. Although there are some associations for the study of pain, none of them are able to give specific referrals.

To find a biofeedback specialist

Upon request (send a self-addressed, stamped envelope with your letter), the Biofeedback Society of America will give you the name of the society in your state that can refer you to a certified biofeedback professional.

Biofeedback Society of America
4301 Owens Street
Wheat Ridge, CO 80033
302-422-8436

To find a hypnotherapist

Contact the nearest hospital-based pain clinic and ask them for a referral. Or you can contact the following societies. All their members meet high standards of professionalism. (They prefer that you write, including a self-addressed, stamped envelope, rather than call.)

Society for Clinical and Experimental Hypnosis
129-A Kings Park Drive
Liverpool, NY 13090
315-652-7299

American Society of Clinical Hypnosis
2250 East Devon Avenue
Suite 336
Des Plaines, IL 60018
312-297-3317

Ontario Society of Clinical Hypnosis
200 St. Clair Avenue West
Suite 402
Toronto, Ontario
Canada M4V 1R1

To find a plastic surgeon for breast reconstruction

Your surgeon or oncologist should be able to recommend a plastic surgeon. Or contact the American Cancer Society or your local medical society. You can also write or call:

American Society of Plastic and Reconstructive Surgeons
Suite 1900
233 N. Michigan Avenue
Chicago, IL 60601
312-856-1834

For free catalogs that list tape recordings of relaxation, imagery, or biofeedback, write to the following three companies:

Psychology Today Tapes
Box 059061
Brooklyn, NY 11205-9061

Among the tapes available from Psych Today are: "Learning to Control Pain" (which focuses on guided imagery); "What Is Hypnosis, and What Can It Do for Me?"; "Two Exercises in Hypnosis"; "Progressive Relaxation"; and "Deep Relaxation and Meditation: An Instructional Cassette."

Guilford Publications, Inc.
200 Park Avenue South
New York, NY 10003

Several excellent audiotapes are available from Guilford. They include these titles: "Passive Muscle Relaxation"; "Personal Enrichment Through Imagery"; "Principles and Practice of Progressive Relaxation: A Teaching Primer"; "Quieting Reflex Training for Adults"; "Relaxation Techniques"; "Relaxation Training Program"; "Self-Transformation Through the New Hypnosis"; and a series of audiotapes, with an accompanying booklet, entitled "Biofeedback Techniques in Clinical Practice."

Carle Medical Communications
510 West Main Street
Urbana, IL 61801

An excellent videotape and audiotape, both entitled "Controlling the Behavioral Side Effects of Chemotherapy" (including exercises in passive relaxation) are available from Carle.

Appendix VII
Further Reading

American Cancer Society, Minnesota Division. *When Mom or Dad Has Cancer.* An illustrated book for young children that discusses the feelings and experiences common to many children of cancer patients.

Anku, Vincent, M.D. *What to Know About the Treatment of Cancer.* Seattle: Madrona Publishers, 1984. A readable book which focuses on the treatment of cancer by chemotherapy.

Belsky, Marvin S., M.D., and Leonard Gross. *How to Choose and Use Your Doctor.* New York: Arbor House, 1979. Some pointers on getting good medical care.

Benson, Herbert, and Miriam Z. Klipper. *The Relaxation Response.* New York: Avon, 1976. A guide to relaxation concepts and techniques.

Berger, Karen, and John Bostich III, M.D. *A Woman's Decision: Breast Care, Treatment, and Reconstruction.* St. Louis, Mo.: C. V. Mosby, 1984. An objective overview of treatments for breast cancer, with a strong focus on reconstruction, and several personal stories.

Bernstein, Joanne E. *Books to Help Children Cope With Separation and Loss,* 2d ed. New York: Bowker, 1983. A comprehensive study of more than six hundred books for young people that deal with various forms of separation and loss. A bibliography of books, chapters in books, and articles for adults is also included.

Blumberg, Rena. *Headstrong: A Story of Conquests and Celebrations . . . Living Through Chemotherapy.* New York: Crown, 1982. The author discusses her own personal experience with breast cancer, and the ways in which she successfully coped with chemotherapy.

Brody, Jane. *Jane Brody's Nutrition Book*. New York: Norton, 1981. Paperback edition, Bantam, 1982. A comprehensive, thorough guide to nutrition and weight control for everyone.

Bruning, Nancy. *Coping with Chemotherapy: How to Take Care of Yourself While Chemotherapy Takes Care of the Cancer*. New York: Doubleday, 1985. A personal but objective and thorough account of every aspect of chemotherapy.

Butler, Robert, and Myrna Lewis. *Love and Sex After Forty*. New York: Harper and Row, 1986. A revised edition of their earlier title, *Love and Sex After Sixty* (1976), this book, like the earlier one, discusses many aspects of sexuality and addresses issues relevant to cancer patients.

Cantor, Robert Chernin. *And a Time to Live: Toward Emotional Well-being During the Crisis of Cancer*. New York: Harper and Row, 1978. Paperback edition, Harper and Row, 1980. This book, by a psychotherapist, explores in full the emotional turmoil that cancer patients and their families face.

Carrera, Michael. *Sex: The Facts, the Acts, and Your Feelings*. New York: Crown, 1981. Good suggestions for those whose sexual performance has been altered by surgery, as well as a full discussion of all aspects of sex and sexuality.

Covell, Mara Brand. *The Home Alternative to Hospitals and Nursing Homes*. New York: Rawson, 1983. Although not specific to cancer patients, much of this book is extremely useful to anyone who is caring for an ill person at home.

Fassler, Joan. *Helping Children Cope: Mastering Stress Through Books and Stories*. New York: The Free Press (Macmillan), 1978. Written by a child psychologist, this book reviews contemporary children's literature to suggest books and stories that can be used to help children deal with various life stresses. Although none of the recommended books deal with cancer in a parent, there are many suggestions for books that deal with separation and loss.

Fiore, Neil A. *The Road Back to Health: Coping With the Emotional Side of Cancer*. New York: Bantam, 1984. The author, a psychotherapist and former cancer patient, focuses on how to deal with being a cancer patient.

Fishman, Joan, R.D., M.S., and Barbara Anrod. *Something's Got to Taste Good: The Cancer Patient's Cookbook*. New York: Andrews and McNeel, Inc. Paperback edition, Signet, 1982. This book gives 170 taste-tempting recipes, carefully selected for ease of preparation, high protein and calorie content.

Glucksberg, Harold, M.D., and Jack W. Singer, M.D. *Cancer Care: A Personal Guide*. Baltimore: Johns Hopkins University Press, 1980. Paperback edition, Scribner's, 1980. Guidebook on types of cancers, treatments, and other special problems of patients.

Greenberger, Monroe E., M.D., and Mary-Ellen Siegel. *What Every Man Should Know About His Prostate*. New York: Walker, 1983. Covers cancer of the prostate, surgical procedures, sex after surgery, and other prostate problems.

Haley, Jay. *Uncommon Therapy*. New York: Norton, 1973. An excellent overview of hypnosis.

Harrington, Geri. *The Health Insurance Fact and Answer Book*. New York: Harper and Row, 1985. An excellent guide to group, individual, disability, and indemnity policies for anyone, including those who have Medicare.

Harrington, Geri. *The Medicare Answer Book*. New York: Harper and Row, 1982. Extremely helpful for anyone who is eligible for Medicare benefits. (Publisher will send free Medicare update to keep you abreast of any major new developments.)

Kelly, Sean F., Ph.D., and Reid J. Kelly, A.C.S.W. *Hypnosis: Understanding How It Can Work For You*. Reading, Mass.: Addison-Wesley, 1985. An introduction for professionals and the general public on the clinical applications of hypnosis. The section on hypnosis and medicine for the control of pain is very useful.

Kushner, Rose. *Alternatives: New Developments in the War on Breast Cancer*. Cambridge, Mass.: Kensington Press, 1984. Formerly published as *Why Me?*, it has been updated from her 1976 and 1982 books in which this medical journalist wrote about her experiences with her own mastectomy and gave important medical information. This new book describes her most recent research in the treatment of recurring breast cancer. The most definitive book on the subject for lay people; it is somewhat technical.

LeShan, Lawrence. *You Can Fight for Your Life: Emotional Factors in the Treatment of Cancer*. New York: Jove paperback (Evans), 1977. How emotions can affect the body's response to cancer.

Margie, Joyce Daly, M.S., and Abby S. Block, M.S., R.D. *Nutrition and the Cancer Patient*. Radnor, Pa.: Chilton, 1983. Background information, specific problems, practical solutions, and recipes are included.

Margolies, Cynthia P., and Kenneth B. McCredie, M.D. *Understanding Leukemia: What It Is, How It's Treated, How to Cope With It.* New York: Scribner's, 1983. Discusses causes, risk factors, treatment, living with leukemia, and research directions.

McKhann, Charles F., M.D. *The Facts About Cancer.* New York: Prentice-Hall, 1981. A helpful book for cancer patients that describes treatments for both children and adults.

Morgan, Susanne. *Coping With a Hysterectomy.* New York: Dial Press, 1981. A helpful book for any woman who has undergone a hysterectomy.

Morra, Marion, and Potts, Eva. *Choices: Realistic Alternatives in Cancer Treatment.* New York: Avon, 1980. Written in question-and-answer format, this comprehensive book covers, in detail, diagnosis, tests, treatments, and side effects.

Mosby Medical Encyclopedia. New York: New American Library, 1985. Based on Mosby's medical and nursing dictionary, this is an excellent home reference book, published in paperback.

Moskowitz, Mark, and Osband, Michael E. *The Complete Book of Medical Tests: A Lifetime Guide for You and Your Family.* New York: Norton, 1984. Good, practical guide to most tests you are likely to have.

Mullen, Barbara Dorr, and Kerry Ann McGinn, R.N. *The Ostomy Book: Living Comfortably With Colostomies, Ileostomies, and Urostomies.* Palo Alto, Calif.: Bull, 1980. Everything the person with an ostomy needs to know.

Nassif, Janet Zhun. *The Home Health Care Solution.* New York: Harper and Row, 1985. A comprehensive guide to every aspect of caring for a sick or elderly person at home. Also includes an outstanding resource guide.

Nierenberg, Judith, R.N., and Florence Janovic. *The Hospital Experience.* New York: Berkley, 1985. An expanded and updated version of their 1978 book, this is a complete guide to understanding and participating in your own care; an essential book for every home library.

Pinckney, Cathey, and Pinckney, Edward, M.D. *The Patient's Guide to Medical Tests.* New York: Facts on File, 1983. Gives complete information on many tests.

Rollin, Betty. *First, You Cry.* New York: Harper and Row, 1976. Paperback edition, New American Library, 1977. A personal, informative story by a news reporter who had a mastectomy.

Rosenbaum, Ernest H., M.D., and Isadora R. Rosenbaum. *A Comprehensive Guide For Cancer Patients and Their Families.* Palo Alto, Calif.: Bull, Special emphasis and detail on stress reduction, nutrition, and physical rehabilitation. (Several sections of this book have been published separately. Write the publisher at Box 208, Palo Alto, CA 94302 for a list of their books on cancer.)

Shipes, Ellen A., and Lehr, Sally T. *Sexual Counseling for Ostomates.* Springfield, Ill.: Charles C. Thomas, 1980. Although addressed to professionals who counsel ostomy patients, this book's common-sense approach makes it useful for patients as well.

Simonton, O. Carl, M.D., Stephanie Matthews-Simonton, and James L. Creighton. *Getting Well Again.* Bantam, 1980. Although according to many cancer experts, the subtitle (A *Step-by-Step, Self-Help Guide to Overcoming Cancer for Patients and Their Families*) is misleading, much in the book is helpful for acquiring positive attitudes, relaxing and managing pain.

Simonton, Stephanie Matthews. *The Healing Family.* New York: Bantam, 1984. Paperback edition, Bantam, 1985. An extremely helpful book for families and those who care about cancer patients. Practical as well as conceptual, it also includes an extensive bibliography.

Snyder, Marilyn. *An Informed Decision: Understanding Breast Reconstruction.* New York: Evans, 1984. The author, a writer and actress, explains breast reconstruction.

Spingarn, Natalie Davis. *Hanging in There: Living Well on Borrowed Time.* Briarcliff Manor, N.Y.: Stein and Day, 1982. Personal narrative by a medical writer who is a cancer patient.

Weisman, Avery, M.D. *Coping With Cancer.* New York: McGraw-Hill, 1979. For health professionals, family, and friends, who want to help cancer patients cope.

Many hospitals, medical centers, and foundations publish fact sheets, pamphlets, and booklets for patients that are available upon request, sometimes for a small fee to cover expenses. Check with your local hospital. Below are the titles of a few useful booklets. Write for further information and current prices.

"Caring at Home for the Broviac-Hickman Catheter: A Guide for Patients and Families." Published by the Department of Nursing, Mount Sinai Medical Center, 1 Gustave L. Levy Place, New York, NY 10029.

"Understanding Chemotherapy: A Guide for Patients and Families." Published by the Department of Neoplastic Diseases, Mount Sinai Medical Center, 1 Gustave L. Levy Place, New York, NY 10029. (Chapters 6 and 12 cover much of the information in this booklet.)

"Radiation Therapy and the Oral Cavity: A Guideline for Patients and Families." Published by the Department of Radiotherapy, Mount Sinai Medical Center, 1 Gustave L. Levy Place, New York, NY 10029.

"Chemotherapy: *Your* Weapon against Cancer." Published by the Chemotherapy Foundation, Inc., 183 Madison Avenue, New York, NY 10016. (Chapters 6 and 12 cover much of the material included in this booklet.)

"Pregnancy and the Woman With an Ostomy"; "Sex and the Female Ostomate"; "Sex and the Male Ostomate"; "Sex, Courtship, and the Single Ostomate"; and many other useful booklets are available from the United Ostomy Association, 2001 West Beverly Boulevard, Los Angeles, CA 90057.

The following excellent booklets and a list of other publications are available free from:

Office of Cancer Communications
National Cancer Institute
Building 31, Room 10A18
Bethesda, MD 20205

"What You Need to Know . . ." A series of useful booklets about different types of cancer; specify cancer site in your request.

"Cancer Treatment." One of a series entitled *Medicine for the Layman*. Overview of cancer growth and treatment.

"Eating Hints: Recipes and Tips for Better Nutrition During Treatment." Well organized booklet for anyone undergoing chemotherapy or radiation therapy.

"Chemotherapy and You: A Guide to Self-Help During Treatment."
Up-to-date information; revised in 1985.

"Radiation Therapy and You: A Guide to Self-Help During Treatment." Also revised in 1985.

"Questions and Answers About Pain Control."

"If You've Thought About Breast Cancer . . ." By Rose Kushner, revised in 1985. A comprehensive booklet that reviews important
issues on detection, diagnosis, treatment, and reconstruction.

"Breast Biopsy: What You Should Know." One- and two-step procedures are fully discussed, along with the implications of diagnosis.

"Mastectomy: A Treatment for Breast Cancer." The various procedures
are discussed.

"Radiation Therapy: A Treatment for Early-Stage Breast Cancer." Ra-
tionale for treatment, as well as the treatment steps involved.

"Breast Reconstruction: A Matter of Choice." Thorough description of
reconstructive plastic surgery following mastectomy.

"Advanced Cancer: Living Each Day." A booklet that discusses the
emotional difficulties and practical realities of dealing with cancer.

"Taking Time: Support for People with Cancer and the People Who
Care About Them." Focuses on the feelings and concerns of cancer patients and of those who care about them.

The NCI will also send you a list of other publications; all of them
are frequently updated, and occasionally new ones are published.

GLOSSARY

Abdomen. The part of the body between the chest and the pelvis. Contains the pancreas, stomach, intestines, kidneys, liver, gallbladder, and other organs.

Abscess. A collection of pus, often resulting in swelling, fever, and pain.

Acquired Immune Deficiency Syndrome (AIDS). A disease caused by an unusual virus that destroys the immune system, leaving the body vulnerable and prone to many diseases, including Kaposi's sarcoma and lymphomas. More than half of those who develop AIDS are homosexual and bisexual men. The rest come from a variety of risk groups, including intravenous-drug users and the sex partners or children of those who have AIDS. A blood test can identify those who have been exposed to the virus.

Acute. Rapidly developing, quick, sudden.

Adenocarcinoma. A cancer whose cells resemble glandular cells when examined under the microscope.

Adenoma. A tumor (benign or malignant) composed of glandular tissue.

Adjuvant chemotherapy. Cancer treatment in which drugs or chemotherapy is given along with surgery or radiation, to attack cancer cells that may be too small to be detected by current diagnostic techniques. Many patients who have solid tumors, which can be surgically removed or destroyed by radiation, also have some microscopic colonies of cancer cells in adjacent areas. Chemotherapy can attack and sometimes destroy these cells *before* they continue to divide and spread.

Alkylating agent. Chemical compound (in drugs) that attaches itself to ever-multiplying cancer cells.

Alopecia. Loss of scalp and body hair.

Alveoli. Tiny air sacs, or clusters, at the end of bronchioles, in the lungs.

Anabolic. Building up strength (appetite, body protein, blood, and muscle).

Analgesic. A drug that can relieve pain without anesthesia or loss of consciousness. Mild analgesics include aspirin and similar products, many of which do not require a prescription.

Anaplastic. Cancer cells that have a "chaotic structure" and are likely to grow quickly (see also *well-differentiated*).

Androgens. Hormones that encourage development and maintenance of male sex characteristics.

Anemia. A condition in which there are fewer than the normal number of red blood cells. Symptoms include shortness of breath, lack of energy, and fatigue.

Anesthesiologist. A physician trained in anesthesia (the administration of anesthetics) and in supervising respiratory and cardiovascular care during surgery and afterward.

Anesthetic. A substance that causes loss of sensation in all or part of the body. Local anesthetic causes lack of sensation. General anesthetic causes loss of consciousness as well as sensation.

Anesthetist. A nurse or other health-care professional with advanced training in the specialty of managing the anesthetic care of patients.

Angiogram. Also called an *arteriogram*, this is a diagnostic radiology test during which dye is introduced into the body so that the vessel structures and arteries leading to various organs are made visible.

Anorexia. Lack or loss of appetite.

Anterior. Front.

Antibiotics. Drugs that can destroy or interfere with the development of infections, bacteria, and other living organisms invading the body. Certain antibiotics are effective against cancer.

Antibody. Part of the body's own defense formed in response to an antigen. Antibodies help defend the body against infection and toxic substance.

Anticoagulant. Medicine used to prevent blood clotting.

Antiemetics. Drugs that prevent or alleviate nausea and vomiting.

Antigen. A substance, foreign to the body's system, that induces resistance to infection or toxic substance.

Antihormones. Drugs that work to block those hormones that stimulate cancer growth.

Antimetabolites. Drugs that act as fraudulent nutrients and "fool" the cells into absorbing them, thereby inhibiting cancer-cell growth.

Antineoplastic. Preventing the development, growth, or spread of cancerous cells.

Antiseptic. Slowing or stopping the growth of microorganisms (germs).

Anxiety. An uncomfortable, often vague, feeling of uneasiness, agitation, or fear, which usually results either from uncertainty or from a consciously or unconsciously anticipated threatened event or outcome.

Artery. A large blood vessel that carries blood from heart to tissues.

Ascites. Accumulation of fluid in the abdominal cavity.

Asymptomatic. Lacking obvious symptoms of disease.

Autoimmunity. A condition in which the body's immune system fights its own tissues and substances.

Axilla. The armpit.

Bacteria. A broad class of one-celled microorganisms, some of which live and feed off other living things. Many, but not all, bacteria are capable of causing disease.

Barium. A metallic element. Milky barium sulfate shows clearly in X-ray pictures, so it is used as a contrast medium in X rays of the digestive tract. It can be swallowed or given through the rectum by means of an enema.

Basal-cell carcinoma. The most common type of skin cancer. It is slow-growing, seldom spreads beneath the skin, and is easily cured, especially if treated promptly. Basal cells are found in small numbers in the lowest part of the epidermis, the outer layer of skin.

BCG (Bacillus Calmette-Guerin). A form of the tuberculosis bacterium used for TB vaccination. Also effective as a stimulant to the immune system, it is frequently given to cancer patients.

Bedsore. See *Decubitus ulcer.*

Benign. Mild or nonmalignant; used to describe an illness or growth. Thus, a benign (or nonmalignant) tumor does not invade or destroy neighboring normal tissue, nor does it spread to other parts of the body.

Betatron. A machine that produces high-energy electrons to treat some cancers that are located deep in the body.

B.I.D. (bis in die). Twice a day.

Bilateral. Pertaining to both sides, as in *bilateral mastectomy.*

Bile. A yellow alkaline fluid secreted by the liver, stored and concentrated in the gallbladder. Bile passes through the common bile duct into the duodenum, where it aids in the digestion of fats.

Biofeedback. A training technique that enables an individual to gain some element of voluntary control over autonomic body functions, such as pulse, skin temperature and brain-wave rhythms. It is based on the principle that a desired response is learned when you receive information or feedback. Biofeedback can help treat pain and such conditions as hypertension and migraine headaches.

Biopsy (used as both verb and noun). Removal and laboratory examination of a small piece of living body tissue to establish or confirm a diagnosis.

Blood-brain barrier. System of tightly meshed cells that help to prevent or slow the passage of chemicals and disease-causing organisms from the blood into the central nervous system.

Blood cells. Cells that make up blood. They are manufactured in the bone marrow and include red blood cells, white blood cells, and platelets.

Blood count. The number of red cells, white cells, and platelets in a given sample of blood. Aids in diagnosis of disease or deficiency.

Blood transfusion. Introduction of whole blood, or just red blood cells, white blood cells, plasma, or platelets, into the circulation to replace lost blood or to correct deficiencies.

Bloodstream. Flowing blood in the circulatory system.

Board-certified specialist. A physician who has received formal training in a medical or surgical specialty and then passed the relevant examination.

Body imaging. Examination techniques that give a picture of the body's interior (e.g., X rays, nuclear scans, CAT scans, ultrasound, thermography, NMR).

Bone marrow. The soft, spongy material found inside the cavities of bone, where many of the important components of the blood are made.

Bone-marrow biopsy and aspiration. Procedure in which a long hollow needle is inserted into the chest or hip bone and a sample of the marrow is suctioned out and then sent to a pathologist for analysis.

Bone-marrow suppression. A decrease in the number of blood cells. This condition may be caused by chemotherapy or radiation, as well as by many medical disorders.

Bone scan. A picture of the bones obtained by injecting a patient with a radioactive chemical that travels to the areas around the bone, highlighting any injury, repair, or destruction. It is an extremely sensitive test, useful in diagnosing cancer that has spread to the bones.

Bone survey. A complete series of X rays of the skeletal system. This survey is useful as a diagnostic aid in detecting cancer.

Bronchi. The large air tubes of the lung, commonly known as the breathing passages.

Bronchioles. The tiny branches of the bronchi.

Bronchoscope. A flexible instrument, inserted through the mouth, that allows a doctor to examine the breathing passages.

BSE. Breast self-examination, allowing a patient to detect early stages of cancer or other disorders.

Carcinoembryonic antigen. A chemical marker that may indicate the presence of cancer cells in laboratory examination of blood.

Carcinogen. A substance known to cause cancer in either animals or humans.

Carcinoma. A cancer that begins in tissues that cover or line the body or internal organs.

Carcinoma in situ. A premalignant growth of cancer that is still confined to the tissue where it originated.

Cardiac. Of or pertaining to the heart.

Cartilage. Tough, firm, flexible tissue covering portions of the bones and freely movable joints.

CAT scan. See *Tomography.*

Catheter. A hollow, flexible tube designed to be passed into a vessel or cavity of the body to withdraw or inject fluids.

Cauterize. To kill tissue with electric current, a heated instrument, or a chemical substance.

Cell. Basic building block of plant and animal tissue. Each cell consists of a small mass of protoplasm, including a nucleus, surrounded by a semipermeable membrane.

Central nervous system (CNS). The brain and spinal cord, which process information and constitute the chief network of coordination and control for the entire body.

Cervix. The necklike portion of the uterus that projects into the vagina.

Chemosurgery. The use of strong drugs, such as zinc chloride, applied directly to the skin to kill cancerous skin cells.

Chemotherapy. Treatment of illness by drugs or medication that can reach all parts of the body; most often used to describe the treatment of cancer by drugs that can interfere with and destroy cancer-cell growth.

Chronic. Continuous or recurring over a long duration. Chronic diseases progress slowly, remain stabile, or flare up repeatedly over a long period of time.

Circulatory system. The network of pathways for blood and nutrient fluids to circulate through the body.

Clinical. Pertaining to the direct study and care of patients, rather than laboratory study.

Clinical disease. A disease that can be recognized by a physician from simple signs and symptoms.

Cobalt-60. A radioactive isotope of the element cobalt. Cobalt-60 machines are used to treat many cancers.

Cocarcinogen. An environmental agent that can act with another to cause cancer.

Colon. The major portion of the large intestine or bowel. It is about five to six feet long. The last five or six inches are the rectum, which leads to the outside of the body.

Colonoscope. A fiber-optic, flexible instrument that is inserted through the rectum to allow a physician to examine the entire length of the colon. Tissue specimens or polyps can be removed during this examination through the colonoscope.

Colorectal cancer. Cancer of the colon and/or rectum.

Colostomy. The surgical procedure in which a new opening for excretion from the colon is created on the surface of the abdomen. Fecal matter is drained into a plastic pouch through this stoma. Procedure may be permanent or temporary. Colostomies are performed for cancer of the lower colon, as well as for some nonmalignant diseases.

Combined chemotherapy. Use of two or more anticancer drugs to treat a patient.

Combined modality treatment. Use of anticancer drugs in combination with surgery and/or radiation therapy. (See also *Adjuvant therapy.*)

Complete blood count (CBC). See *Blood count.*

Computerized tomography. See *Tomography.*

Conization. Surgical removal of a cone-shaped piece of tissue from the cervix and cervical canal. Used for both diagnosis and treatment.

Contraindicated. Prohibiting the use of a certain drug or procedure.

Contrast medium. A dye injected or gradually flowed into a vein to highlight internal structures for visualization through X rays and other body-imaging techniques.

Cordotomy. The surgical procedure in which nerves are cut in the spinal cord to eliminate excessive pain.

Cortisone. Synthetic forms of steroid hormones that occur naturally in the body; used to treat inflammatory conditions and diseases, including cancer.

Cryosurgery. Surgery that makes use of an extremely low-temperature probe.

CT scan. See *Tomography.*

Curative treatment. Treatment designed to cure.

Curettage. A surgical procedure in which material is scraped and removed from an organ, cavity, or other surface.

Cyst. A closed sac in or under skin, containing fluid or semisolid material.

Cystectomy. Surgical removal of the bladder.

Cystoscope. A lighted instrument that is passed through the urethra and into the bladder for examination of the bladder interior.

Cytology. Examination of a smear of tissue or cells from the body.

Cytotoxic. Poisonous to cells.

Decubitus ulcer. Ulceration or sore that may develop from constant pressure, often occurring in patients who are in bed for long periods of time. Commonly called a bedsore.

Depression. Emotional state characterized by feelings of sadness, despair, and discouragement, which may be either appropriate or out of proportion to reality.

Dermal. Pertaining to skin.

Diagnosis. The process of determining the nature of a disease so that it can be properly treated.

Differential count. The density of various types of white cells in blood.

Differentiation modifiers. Experimental drugs that seek to change cancer cells to normal cells without affecting surrounding normal cells.

Digestive tract. The organs and glands of the system through which food passes from mouth to esophagus, stomach, and intestines. Glands secrete enzymes, which break down food substances for absorption into the bloodstream before carrying waste to intestines for excretion.

Diuretics. Drugs that increase the elimination of water and salts from the body, thus increasing elimination of urine.

Dosimetrist. A health professional who works with the physician in calculating the proper dosage of radiation for cancer treatment.

DRGs. Abbreviation for diagnostic-related groups, a system that classifies patients by age, diagnosis, procedures, and treatment, producing a number of different categories used in predicting the use of hospital resources, including length of stay. Medical-insurance companies reimburse hospitals a fixed fee for each patient who has been so classified.

Drug-resistant. Able to resist the curative effects of a drug. Sometimes cancer cells can develop this property over a period of treatment, rendering a certain drug useless.

Duodenum. The first part of the small intestine.

Dysplasia. Abnormal development.

-ectomy. A suffix meaning "surgical removal" (of body part specified in preceding part of word, as in *tonsil*lectomy).

Edema. An abnormal swelling caused by the accumulation of fluid in tissues.

Effusion. The escape of fluid from blood vessels into a body cavity.

Electrocardiogram (EKG or ECG). A graphic record or tracing of the actions of various portions of the heart. The instrument used for the recording is an electrocardiograph, and the graphic record it produces is used in the diagnosis of heart disease.

Electrocoagulation. The surgical procedure in which a needle or snare is used to destroy tissues. Also called *galvanocautery.*

Electrodessication. A form of electrosurgery in which tissue is destroyed by burning with an electric spark. Also called *fulguration.*

Electroencephalogram. A painless diagnostic test that yields a graphic record measuring electrical activity in various parts of the brain.

Electrolytes. Compounds that provide the necessary environment for cells of the body. They include calcium, potassium, sodium, and chloride.

Electrons. Negatively charged particles of atoms. Radiotherapy often makes
·use of electron beams.
Electrosurgery. Surgery performed with various electrical instruments that operate on high-frequency electrical current (e.g., electrocoagulation, electrodessication).
Endocrine system. The network of glands and tissues that secrete hormones
directly into the bloodstream. The endocrine system includes the brain,
ovaries, testicles, kidneys, adrenals, thyroid gland, pituitary gland, pancreas, the stomach lining, and the intestines. Secretions from the endocrine glands affect various processes throughout the body, such as
metabolism and growth.
Endometrium. The lining of the uterus.
Endorphins. The body's own morphine, which can be released by placebos
and various metabolic processes, having a relaxing or euphoric effect.
Endoscope. Any rigid or flexible tubular instrument that allows a physician to
examine the body interior for abnormalities so that he may also remove
them or take tissue samples. An endoscope can be inserted through the
mouth, rectum, vagina, urethra, or any other natural body opening; or
it may be inserted through a surgical incision. (See also *Fiber optic*,
Bronchoscope, Cystoscope, Sigmoidoscope, Proctoscope, Colonoscope.)
Endoscopy. Any diagnostic test performed with an endoscope.
Epidermoid carcinoma. A lung cancer whose cells resemble those of the skin.
It is also called squamous-cell carcinoma.
Esophagus. The narrow muscular digestive tube leading to the stomach.
Estrogens. A general name for female sex hormones, formed in the ovaries in
women, and in the adrenal glands in both men and women. They are
responsible for the development and maintenance of the female repro-
ductive tract and secondary sex characteristics of the female. Synthetic
estrogens are used in the treatment of prostatic and breast cancer.
Estrogen-receptor assay (ER assay). A laboratory test that can establish if a
breast cancer is estrogen-dependent.
Estrogen receptors. Proteins that carry estrogen, increasing functioning
ability.
Excision. Surgical removal of tissue or a body part, including any cancerous
growth.
External radiation. Radiotherapy using a machine from which radiation is
directed toward the diseased part of the body.

Fallopian tubes. The pair of tubes, one on each side of the uterus, that transport the egg from the ovaries to the uterus.
Fiber. The stringy or coarse part of certain fruits, vegetables, and grains; often
referred to as bulk or roughage. High-fiber, low-fat diets are considered
helpful in lowering one's chances of developing cancer.
Fiber optics. The process in which flexible tubelike instruments, using glass
or plastic fibers to transmit and bend light and reflect a magnified image,
can be inserted into the body to make visible (and biopsy, if indicated)
otherwise inaccessible areas of the body. (See *Endoscope*.)
Fluoroscope. A radiological device that shows an immediate projection of an

X-ray image on a fluorescent screen. It looks something like a television screen displaying a "motion-picture X ray."

Folic-acid antagonist. A chemical compound that can destroy cancer cells.

Follicle. A pouchlike depression in the skin, formed before birth, from which hair grows. Chemotherapy can temporarily damage follicles, causing hair loss. Radiotherapy can temporarily or even permanently have this effect.

Fulguration. See *Electrodessication*.

Gallium scan. A nuclear scan that can visualize rapidly dividing cells and detect lymph-node involvement. A small amount of gallium-67 is injected into the veins prior to this test.

Galvanocautery. See *Electrocoagulation*.

Gamma rays. A type of radiation that is used to treat cancer. When source of ray is a radioactive substance, ray is called a gamma ray. X rays are an example.

Gastroenterologist. A physician who specializes in diseases of the digestive tract, including the stomach, intestines, gallbladder, and bile duct.

Gastrointestinal (GI). Relating to the digestive tract, including mouth, stomach, intestines, and rectum.

Genitourinary (GU). Referring to the genital and urinary systems.

Gland. An organ that selectively removes material from bloodstream and converts it to a new substance, which may be recirculated through the bloodstream for a specific function or excreted.

Guaiac test. See *Hemoccult*.

Gynecologist. A physician who specializes in female physiology, endocrinology, and reproductive diseases.

Gynecomastia. Excessive enlargement and development of breasts in men.

Hematocrit (Hct). A test to determine the percentage of the volume of blood taken up by cells. A "low" hematocrit indicates anemia.

Hematologist. A physician who specializes in problems of the blood and bone marrow. Many hematologists also specialize in treating cancer patients.

Hematuria. Any condition in which the urine contains blood or red blood cells.

Hemoccult. An important hidden-blood detection test. Samples of stool are taken by the patient at home after a few days on a restricted diet. A doctor analyzes the results. A similar "do-it-yourself" kit is available in drugstores. Traces of blood in the stool may suggest the possibility of cancer of the rectum or colon long before obvious symptoms appear. Also called a *Guaiac test*.

Hemoglobin (Hgb). A protein-iron compound in the blood that carries oxygen from lungs to tissues and removes carbon dioxide from cells.

Hodgkin's disease. A form of cancer affecting lymphatic and related tissue.

Hormone. A chemical product formed in one part of the body (usually endocrine glands) that is carried in the blood to other parts. When hormones are secreted into body fluids, they have a specific effect on other organs.

Hormonotherapy. The treatment of cancer with hormones, usually in conjunction with other methods, such as surgery or chemotherapy.

Hospice. A place or program in which a terminally ill patient can maintain a satisfactory life-style until death. Most hospice programs are multidisciplinary and include physicians, nurses, social workers, and others who aid and support patient and family and also help family give support to patient.

Hyperalimentation. The intravenous administration of greater-than-optimum amounts of nutrients. (See also *Total parenteral nutrition*.)

Hyperplasia. An increase in the number of cells in a tissue or organ, not necessarily related to cancer.

Hyperthermia. An experimental cancer treatment in which heat is applied to either the entire body or the tumor.

Hypnosis. A passive, trancelike state resembling normal sleep, during which perception and memory are altered, permitting the person to respond to suggestions. Suggestions for the posthypnotic period can also be made during hypnosis.

Hypodermic. Underneath the skin; refers to injection through the skin into underlying fat.

Ileostomy. The surgical procedure in which an artificial opening is created between the small bowel (ileum) and the abdominal wall, through which fecal matter is passed. Procedure may be permanent or temporary. Ileostomies are performed for cancer of the large bowel as well as for some nonmalignant diseases.

Immune response. The body's defensive reaction against infection, producing antibodies or activating lymphocytes to destroy foreign substances such as chemicals, particles, microorganisms, and even cancer cells.

Immunity. The body's ability to resist or overcome infection. This can be inborn or acquired (naturally or artificially), temporary or of long duration.

Immunotherapy. Treatment directed at producing immunity or resistance to a disease or condition.

Infiltration. Passage of cells or fluid into areas where they are usually not present.

Inflammation. Warmth, redness, or swelling, as a reaction to the presence or growth of bacteria in the body.

Infusion. Introduction of fluid slowly or continuously into circulatory system by means of gravity flow.

Infusion pump. An apparatus designed to deliver measured amounts of a drug through injection over a period of time. Some can be implanted surgically.

Injection. Forcing a liquid into the body by means of a syringe. Any medication, including those used in chemotherapy, may be given in one of these ways:

    IM (Intramuscular): within or into a muscle.

    IC (Intracavitary): within or into a body cavity.

    IT (Intrathecal): within or into the spinal area.

IV (Intravenous): within or into a vein.

SC (Subcutaneous): just under the skin.

Insulin. A pancreatic hormone secreted into the blood. Regulates the amount of sugar in blood.

Interferon. Cellular proteins that inhibit the intracellular replication of a broad range of viruses. This chemical substance is naturally released by the body in response to viral infections. Can be synthesized.

Internal radiation. The implantation of a radioactive substance into the body close to area that requires radiotherapy.

Interstitial radiation. The implanting of a radioactive substance directly into the tissue requiring radiotherapy.

Intracavitary radiation. The implantation of a radioactive source into a body cavity, such as the vagina or prostate.

Intravenous drip. Technique in which a patient receives a substance through a needle connected to a plastic tube that leads to a liquid-filled bottle suspended from a pole. Substance can be dripped in gradually at a predetermined rate.

Intravenous pyelogram (IVP). A series of X rays taken after the intravenous injection of dye into the patient's bloodstream. These pictures outline the urinary bladder, ureters, and kidneys. Also called intravenous urography.

Invasion. The spread of cancer cells from the original site into surrounding tissues or organs.

Irradiation. See *Radiation*.

Isotope. See *Radionuclide*.

Kidneys. The two bean-shaped organs located on either side of the spinal column. Blood passes through them, and the impurities that are removed there dissolve and form urine.

Laparoscopy. A test in which a small incision is made into the abdomen and a lighted tube is inserted, allowing the doctor to examine the ovaries and abdominal contents and to remove a piece of tissue for biopsy.

Laparotomy. An incision through the wall of the abdomen.

Large-cell carcinoma. Lung cancer characterized by large cells that do not resemble the cells of other types of lung cancer.

Laryngectomy. Surgical removal of the larynx.

Larynx. The upper portion of windpipe, containing the vocal cords. Also called the voice box.

Laser. An acronym for *light amplification by stimulated emission of radiation*. A laser beam is an extremely concentrated source of light that gives off so much heat it can destroy anything in its path.

Lesion. A mass of cells, which may be solid, semisolid (cystic), inflammatory, benign, or malignant. Term also applies to a lump or abscess.

Leukemia. Cancers of the blood and circulatory system, usually arising in the bone marrow.

Leukopenia. A decrease in the manufacture of white blood cells.

Linear accelerator. A highly accurate machine that creates and uses high energy and radiation to treat cancer.

Liver. The large glandular organ that secretes bile and causes important changes in many substances contained in blood.

Lobe. A portion of the lung.

Lobectomy. Surgical removal of one lobe of a lung.

Localized. Remaining at the site of origin (refers to cancer cells).

Lumbar puncture. Removal of fluid from the spine. Also called *spinal tap.*

Lymph. A clear, transparent, watery, sometimes faintly yellowish liquid containing white blood cells and some red blood cells. It travels through the lymph system removing bacteria from tissues, transporting fat from intestines, and supplying lymphocytes to blood.

Lymph nodes or glands. Structures throughout the body that contain lymph. They also act as a defense, triggering an immune response to cancer as well as to bacteria. Often the first area to which cancer spreads.

Lymphangiogram. A diagnostic test to visualize lymph glands deep in the abdomen.

Lymphatic system. The interconnected circulatory system of spaces and vessels that carry lymph throughout the body.

Lymphedema. Swelling that results from obstruction of lymphatic vessels or nodes.

Lymphocytes. Colorless cells produced in lymphoid organs such as the lymph nodes, spleen, and thymus. Lymphocytes fight infection.

Lymphoma. Cancer arising in the spleen or lymph glands.

Lymphosarcoma. Cancer arising in lymphatic tissue.

Malignant. Cancerous.

Malignant tumor. A growth of cancer cells.

Mammogram. A low-dose X ray directed at the breasts to reveal their inner structure; can detect breast cancer even before it can be felt on examination.

Mastectomy. Surgical removal of a breast.

Maxillofacial prosthesis. Artificial replacement for missing parts of the face.

Mediastinotomy. Surgical exploration of the mediastinum, the area between the lungs and the breastbone.

Megavoltage therapy. High-energy radiotherapy that is measured in millions of volts. Can be precisely directed to the area requiring radiotherapy.

Melanoma. A skin cancer that often begins in a pigmented mole. Unchecked, it can invade lymph nodes and organs.

Meningoma. A common benign tumor that begins in the tissues lining the brain.

Metastasis. Shifting, spreading, colonization, or seeding of an original cancerous tumor to form growths or tumors in other parts of the body. It is usually transplanted through the bloodstream or lymph channels.

Metastatic lesion. A small patch of malignant tissue or tumor that has spread from the original site of cancer, however remote.

Mitotic inhibitors. Drugs that act to prevent cancer cells from dividing (mitosis), thus interfering with the process by which they grow and replicate themselves.

Modality. Method of treatment. The three chief modalities for treatment of cancer are surgery, radiotherapy, and chemotherapy.

Monoclonal antibodies. Antibodies, formed by cloning (artificially replicating) fused cells, that form antigens. A potential treatment for cancer.

Mucositis. See *Stomatitis.*

Mucous membrane. Thin sheets of tissue that cover or line various parts of body, such as mouth, digestive tract, respiratory passages, and genitourinary tract.

Multimodality therapy. The use of several methods to treat a disease. Treatments may be given concurrently, or one may follow another.

Myeloma. A cancer that forms tumors composed of cells normally found in bone marrow. It often forms in ribs, vertebrae, pelvic bones.

Narcotic. An analgesic drug that is derived from opium or produced synthetically. Narcotic drugs act by binding to opiate receptors in the central nervous system.

Neoplasm. A tumor, abnormal growth, or swelling of tissue. It can be either benign or malignant, usually the latter.

Nephrectomy. Surgical removal of a kidney.

Neuroblastoma. A malignant tumor of the nervous system, composed of immature nerve cells.

Neurologist. A physician who specializes in disorders of the nervous system.

Neuroma. A benign tumor composed of nerve cells and/or nerve fibers.

Neurosurgeon. A physician who performs surgery on the brain, spinal cord, or peripheral nerves.

Neutron-beam radiation. A radiation technique effective against otherwise radio-resistant cells.

NG. Nasogastric.

NMR. See Nuclear magnetic resonance.

Nodule. A small mass of tissue or tumor, generally malignant.

NPO (Non per os). Nothing by mouth.

Nuclear magnetic resonance (NMR). A new diagnostic technique that produces a body-section image and can detect dead or degenerating cells, blockage of blood flow, and cancer.

Nuclear medicine. A specialty encompassing training in the newer nuclear imaging tests. Physicians who specialize in nuclear medicine are also trained in internal medicine, pathology, and radiology.

Nuclear scan. A diagnostic test that makes use of a small amount of radioactive trace compounds.

Obstruction. A blockage of a natural passageway.

Occupational therapist. A trained health professional who uses purposeful specific activity with people whose ability to function independently is limited for any number of reasons, including physical injury or illness. His or her goal is to help people become more independent in activities of daily living.

-oma. A tumor (e.g., melanoma, lymphoma, neuroma).

Oncogenes. Cancer genes, which may be linked with changes in chromosomes, altering normal genes so that they become cancerous.

Oncologist. A physician especially trained to treat cancer. *Medical oncologists* usually treat patients with chemotherapy and often coordinate all the treatment of the cancer patient. *Surgical oncologists* specialize in the surgical treatment of cancer patients. *Radiation oncologists* specialize in the use of radiotherapy on cancer patients.

Oncology. The study, science, and treatment of neoplasms and tumors.

Oophorectomy. Surgical removal of one or both ovaries.

Orally. By mouth.

Orchidectomy. The surgical removal of one or both testicles. Sometimes performed for cancer of the prostate or testicles. Also called *orchiectomy.*

Organ. A strutural collection of tissues and cells that together perform one or more particular functions (e.g., liver, spleen, digestive organs, reproductive organs).

Orthopedist. A physician who treats and/or performs surgery associated with problems of the skeletal system, its joints, muscles, and associated structures.

Orthovoltage. Radiation treatment with less energy than is delivered by the megavoltage equipment that is now used for many cancers. Still used for certain malignancies.

Ostomy. Any surgical procedure that constructs an artificial opening, called a *stoma.* Procedures are named for the location of the ostomy.

Otolaryngologist. A physician who treats and performs surgery on the ear, nose, mouth, and throat.

Ovaries. The pair of female organs responsible for production of eggs and female sex hormones. They are located on each side of the lower abdomen, beside the uterus.

Palliative treatment. Treatment that is not aimed at cure, but makes a patient feel better, relieving symptoms, pain, or discomfort from a disease.

Palpation. A technique in which the physician uses hands, rather than instruments, to examine organs to determine texture, size, consistency, and location.

Pancreas. The large gland that stretches across the abdominal wall behind the stomach. It secretes various substances, such as digestive fluids and the hormone insulin.

Pancytopenia. Decrease of white blood cells, red blood cells, and platelets.

Pap (Papanicolaou) smear. A diagnostic test that screens for cancer of the uterus and cervix by microscopic examination of cells collected during a routine pelvic examination. Efficiently detects early cervical cancer, but picks up only 50 percent of endometrial cancers.

Papillary tumor. A small mushroom-shaped tumor with a stem attached to the inner lining of a body cavity.

Paracentesis. A procedure in which fluid is removed from the abdomen.

Paresthesia. Skin sensation of burning, prickling, tingling, itching, numbing, usually in fingers or toes.

Pathology. The part of medicine that deals with the results of disease, particularly as seen in cell, organ, and tissue changes.

Pelvic examination. Examination of the organs of the pelvis (the female reproductive organs and rectum).

PET. See *Positron emission tomography.*

Pharmacology. Study of the preparation, properties, uses, and actions of drugs, including their absorption, distribution throughout the body, and excretion.

Pharynx. The upper part of the throat, which serves as a passageway for the respiratory and digestive tracts.

Phase I. Initial study of very new and still experimental drugs.

Phase II. Further study of drugs, usually only available on limited basis, to test their effectiveness.

Phase III. Further study of drugs at medical centers to determine optimum dose as well as further information on safety and effectiveness.

Phlebitis. Inflammation of a vein.

Physical Therapist. A trained professional who assists in the examination, testing, and treatment of people who are temporarily or permanently physically disabled. An important part of the medical team for many cancer patients whose disease or treatment has in some way limited their movement. Physical therapists use special exercises, applications of heat or cold, sonar waves, and other techniques.

Placebo. An inactive substance prescribed as if it were an effective dose of a needed medication.

Plasma. The watery, colorless portion of lymph and blood that contains various elements necessary for normal body functioning, including platelets, proteins, and minerals.

Platelet. An irregularly shaped disk in the bloodstream that aids in clotting. A reduction in platelets can lead to bleeding or bruising.

Platelet count. The number of platelets per cubic millimeter of blood.

Pleural tap. See *Thoracentesis.*

PO (Per os). By mouth.

Polyp. A benign mass of tissue growth protruding from a mucous membrane (e.g., nasal polyps, rectal polyps). Some polyps are precancerous, and for this reason it is often recommended that they be removed and evaluated by a pathologist.

Positron emission tomography (PET). A diagnostic test that takes pictures of the chemical activity of the brain after radioactive glucose has been injected into the body.

Posterior. In the back or rear.

PR (per rectum). Rectally.

Primary tumor. Original tumor. Even if tumor spreads, forming a secondary or metastatic tumor, it is still referred to by the name of its primary or original tumor. (Thus, breast cancer that has spread to a lung is still called breast cancer.)

PRN (pro re nata). As often as necessary.

Proctoscope. An instrument used to examine the rectum and anus (see also *Sigmoidoscope*).

Progesterone. A natural hormone used in the treatment of various menstrual disorders and related problems.

Progesterone-receptor assay. A test that indicates whether or not a breast cancer is dependent on female hormones for nourishment.

Prognosis. The doctor's forecast of the progress and probable outcome of a disease.

Prophylaxis. Prevention of, or protection against, a disease or its complications.

Prostate. The male gland that surrounds the urethra, next to the inner wall of the rectum, directly below the bladder. It secretes fluid that forms part of semen.

Prostatectomy. Surgical removal of all or part of the prostate gland. A *total prostatectomy* is the removal of the entire prostate gland and the capsule in which it is enclosed. A *retropubic* or *suprapubic prostatectomy* is the removal of all or part of the prostate gland through an incision in the abdomen. A *transurethral resection of the prostate (TUR or TURP)* is the surgical removal of all or part of the prostate gland by means of passing an instrument through the penis and urethra to cut away tissue in the prostate gland. These procedures are sometimes performed for cancer of the prostate.

Prosthesis. An artificial replacement for a missing part of the body.

Proteins. Compounds that are a main component of all animal tissue. The major source of building material for muscles, blood, skin, hair, nails, and the intestines. Occur naturally in meat, eggs, milk, and some grains.

Protocol. A written, predetermined treatment plan that specifies what drugs a patient will receive, in what doses, and how frequently. Scientific study designed to determine the most effective treatment for a specific type of cancer.

Psychiatrist. A physician who specializes in the branch of medicine that deals with the causes, treatment, and prevention of mental, emotional, and behavioral disorders. Some psychiatrists specialize in the relationship between physical disease and emotions, and may have an expertise in the emotional problems common to cancer patients.

Pulmonary. Of or pertaining to the lungs or respiratory system.

qid (quater in die). Four times a day.

qn (quaque nox). Every night.

q2h (quaque secunda hora). Every two hours.

q4h (quaque quarta hora). Every four hours.

Rad. Abbreviation for *radiation-absorbed doses;* the unit of measurement for radiation.

Radiation. The emission of energy from one source or center. In medicine, the rays emitted are used for purposes of treatment or diagnosis.

Radiation oncologist. See *Radiotherapist.*

Radiation physicist. A professional who computes proper radiation doses for therapy.

Radiation therapy. A treatment using high-energy radiation from X-ray machines, or electrons from a cobalt, betatron, or other machine.

Radioactive. Emitting radiant energy.

Radioactive implant. Radioactive material (wire, needle, capsule, or container) placed inside the body near the cancer. This implant can deliver a high dose of radiation to the malignant area while sparing the surrounding normal tissue.

Radiocurable. Curable by radiation therapy alone.

Radioisotope. A radioactive isotope (a chemical element) used for therapeutic and diagnostic purposes.

Radiologist. A physician who specializes in various kinds of body imaging, most of which make use of radioactive substances.

Radiopaque. Opaque to radiation. Any contrast medium that is taken internally to block X rays so that body structures show up clearly on an X-ray film is radiopaque. (Barium is an example.)

Radioresistant. Resistant to the effects of radiotherapy (refers to cancers that will not always shrink under radiation).

Radiosensitive. Cancer that usually shrinks as a result of radiotherapy.

Radiotherapist. A physician who is specially trained in the use of radiation therapy to treat patients.

Recovery room. A special area in a hospital where patients are held after surgery, prior to returning to their hospital room. They remain here until they are awake and able to respond. Nurses with special training monitor their vital signs.

Rectum. The end portion of the large intestine extending from the sigmoid colon to the anal canal.

Recurrence. The return of cancer symptoms or tumor (may or may not be expected). A tumor may recur in the site of origin or elsewhere, having metastasized. (See also *Relapse*.)

Red blood cells (rbc). Small, disk-shaped cells that float in blood and contain hemoglobin. They are responsible for the color of the blood, the transport of oxygen to the tissues, and the removal of carbon dioxide from tissues. A reduction in red blood cells can lead to anemia.

Red blood count (RBC). The number of red blood cells per cubic centimeter.

Regional involvement. Spread of cancer from its primary site to adjacent areas.

Regional perfusion. Chemotherapy directed with a catheter to a limited area of the body to destroy cancer tissue with minimal damage to normal tissue.

Regression. Shrinkage and subsidence of cancer growth.

Relapse. A return of symptoms after improvement had been noted.

Remission. The disappearance of signs and symptoms of cancer.

Renal. Pertaining to the kidneys.

Resect. To cut off or excise a segment of a body part or organ.

Resectable. Amenable to surgical removal.

Respiratory. Referring to the breathing system, including windpipe, bronchial tubes, and lungs.

Rhizotomy. The surgical procedure in which a nerve is severed close to the spinal cord, preventing the transmission of pain to the pain-perception area of the brain.

Right-atrial catheter. A hollow, flexible tube that is inserted directly into a patient's circulatory system to provide a pathway for nutrients, medications, chemotherapy, fluid, and/or blood products. Blood samples for tests may also be obtained through this catheter without discomfort.

RT. Radiation therapy.

Rx. Treatment.

Saline solution. Solution of salt and water.

Sarcoma. Cancer that originates in bones and from tissues that connect or lie between organs and skin.

Scans. Computerized pictures of an organ or body part, such as the bones, liver, or brain. Radioactive substances are sometimes injected into the patient prior to the scan. These concentrate in the sections of the body to be scanned, thereby aiding visualization.

Seminal vesicles. Two folded glandular structures that lie against the lower rear bladder wall in men. The secretions of the seminal vesicles form part of semen.

Septic. Infected.

Shunt. A tube or other device implanted in the body to redirect the flow of a body fluid from one cavity or vessel to another.

Side effects. Temporary reaction to drugs or radiation other than the expected curative effects. There is *no* relationship between side effects and treatment effectiveness.

Sigmoidoscope. An instrument that is inserted through the rectum to examine the lower portion of the colon. It is a foot-long semirigid tube often used in routine checkups on people over the age of fifty. The lower one third of the colon is made visible during this test. For a more complete examination a colonoscope must be used. Sometimes also called a *proctosigmoidoscope.* (See also *Proctoscope* and *Colonoscope.*)

Small-cell carcinoma. Lung cancer whose cells are small and round; also called *oat-cell carcinoma.*

Small intestine. The part of the digestive tract that extends from the stomach to the large intestine.

Social worker. A trained professional who strives to enhance and maintain psychosocial functioning of individuals, families, and small groups. Hospital social workers assess the home situation, finances, and community resources as well as social and emotional factors that are specifically related to the patient's medical condition, and then take action to help resolve any problems. They provide counseling and psychotherapy to the patient and family, and help with discharge plans.

Sonogram. A computer picture that uses ultrasound (high-frequency sound waves) to examine position, form, and function of anatomical structures. The vibrations or waves are sent through various parts of the body to create a picture of various layers of the inside of the body. A sonogram is the record of ultrasound tests.

Spinal tap. See *Lumbar puncture.*

Spleen. An organ, near the stomach, that performs various functions such as blood production and storage, destruction of old or damaged red blood cells and platelets. Can become enlarged in various cancers.

Sputum. Material composed of mucus, cellular debris, microorganisms, coughed up from lungs and expectorated through mouth. Sputum can contain blood or pus.

Sputum test. Laboratory examination of sputum for diagnosis of many illnesses, including lung cancer.

Squamous-cell carcinoma. A slow-growing cancer. When found on the skin, it is easily cured when treated promptly.

Stabilization. The state in which a disease or tumor remains the same, neither shrinking, growing, nor spreading.

Staging. Careful evaluation to determine extent of a patient's disease.

Steroids. Chemical substances consisting of many hormones, vitamins, and other substances. There are natural and synthetic derivatives of steroids. Often used as cancer treatment.

Stilbesterol. A synthetic female hormone, frequently given to patients with cancer of the prostate.

Stoma. A surgically created artificial opening of an internal organ to the surface of the body. A stoma of intestines or urinary tract results in elimination of wastes through abdomen wall. A stoma of respiratory tract results in the passage of air through the neck instead of mouth and nose.

Stomatitis. Inflammation of the mucous membranes of the mouth, often resulting in sores in the mouth. Also called *mucositis*.

Subclinical. Refers to an illness or disease that is so mild, or at such an early stage, that it produces no visible symptoms and cannot be easily detected.

Superior vena cava. The second-largest vein in the body, which returns blood from the upper half of the body to the right atrium of the heart.

Supine. Lying face up.

Suture. A surgical stitch bringing together two surfaces.

Systemic disease. A disease that affects the whole body rather than just one portion of it.

TENS. See *Transcutaneous electric nerve stimulation*.

Terminal disease. An illness from which no remission or improvement is expected. Despite stabilization, a patient may be defined as terminal, although not near or approaching death. Some authorities use the term only for cases in which death is expected within three months; others reserve its use for more imminent situations.

Thermography. A heat picture made with heat-sensitive film, which uses infrared light radiated by the skin to detect temperature differences in tissues that may indicate an infection or cancer.

Thoracentesis. Removal of fluid from the pleural space surrounding the lungs. Also called *pleural tap*.

Thoracotomy. Major surgical procedure in which an incision is made in the chest and a lung to examine the lung for cancer or other disease.

Thorax. The cage of bone and cartilage containing the lungs and heart.

Thrombocytopenia. Abnormal condition in which platelet count is decreased, owing to various causes such as cancer or immune response to a drug. Can be caused by chemotherapy.

Thyroid gland. A gland, in the front of the neck, that produces the hormone thyroxine, essential to normal body growth in infancy and childhood. Part of the endocrine system.

TID (ter in die). Three times a day.

Titrate. To analyze a medicated solution and find the smallest dose of a drug necessary to bring about the desired effect. To relieve pain, a solution may be "titrated up" as needed. In chemotherapy, titration requires a balance that will keep desired antitumor effects to a maximum and toxic effects to a minimum.

Tolerance. An individual's level of resistance to desired or undesired effects of a drug.

Tomography. A diagnostic technique using computers and X rays to obtain a highly detailed image of a section of the body being studied. Tomograms usually make use of contrast dye.

Topically. Applied to the surface of the body.

Total parenteral nutrition (TPN). The administration of nutrients through a catheter directly into the superior vena cava. TPN allows continuous and total replacement of nutrient needs at a slow, steady rate, and is used when feeding by mouth does not provide adequate amounts of essential nutrients.

Toxic reaction. Serious side effects or reactions, some of which are potentially dangerous.

Trachea. The tube leading from the back of the mouth down to the bronchial tubes, conveying air to the lungs. Also called the *windpipe*.

Tracheotomy (or tracheostomy). A surgical opening in the windpipe through the front of the neck, to allow air to enter lungs and mucus to be suctioned out.

Transcutaneous electric nerve stimulation (TENS). A procedure in which mild electrical stimulation to the skin is used to relieve chronic pain.

Transillumination. Procedure in which a powerful light is placed next to a suspicious area on skin to increase visualization.

Tumor. A purposeless swelling or enlargement in the body. Can be either benign (noncancerous) or malignant (cancerous). Cancer cells often cluster to form a mass or tumor.

Tumor board. An official committee, in a hospital or community, composed of physicians including medical, radiation, and surgical oncologists; pathologists; and sometimes other health professionals. They review cases of cancer from the hospital and elsewhere, and make recommendations concerning further diagnosis or treatment. A patient can ask his own physician to submit his case to a tumor board.

TUR. See *Prostatectomy*.

Ultrasound. See *Sonogram*.

Unilateral. On one side of body only.

Ureter. The long, narrow tube through which urine passes from the kidney to the bladder.

Urethra. The muscular canal through which urine passes from the bladder out of the body. In men, seminal fluid passes through the urethra as well.

Urinary diversion. See *Urostomy*.

Urologist. A physician who specializes in the diagnosis and treatment of diseases of the male genitourinary tract and female urinary tract.

Urostomy. Procedure in which an artificial bladder is created to store urine following the removal of the bladder. The ureters are disconnected from the bladder and are joined to the end of a small segment of the ileum (part of the small intestine). This segment of the ileum is converted into a conduit, or tube, and is brought through the wall of the abdomen near the navel, where it forms an opening called a *stoma*. This enables urine to flow out of the body. A flat pouch is placed over the stoma to collect urine. Also called *urinary diversion*.

Uterus. Female organ of reproduction, also known as womb, in which fetus develops. The uterus has two parts; a body and cervix. The latter extends into the vagina.

Vein. A blood vessel that carries blood from tissues to the heart and lungs.

Venipuncture. The injection of a needle into a vein to take blood or give medication.

Vital signs. Temperature, pulse, respiratory rate, and blood pressure.

Vitamins. Compounds that, in small quantities, are essential for normal growth, maintenance, and functioning of the body. Vitamins are obtained from well-balanced diets, but many healthy people need supplements. Cancer patients frequently need additional supplements, but they should *only* be taken in consultation with an oncologist. Some vitamins, such as folic acid, can interfere with chemotherapy. Vitamin therapy is not a proven substitute for surgery, chemotherapy, or radiotherapy for the treatment of cancer.

Well-differentiated. A term used to describe cancer cells which are well structured and likely to be slow-growing.

White blood cells (wbc). Several blood-cell types, containing no hemoglobin, that are active in response to disease, immunity, and medication. White blood cells are about one third larger than red blood cells, and they act against infection.

White blood count (WBC). The number of white blood cells per cubic centimeter.

Workup. The combined results of a medical examination and tests, often done in a hospital, to arrive at a diagnosis and complete medical picture of the patient.

X ray. A gamma ray used to make diagnostic pictures of the body interior; one of those pictures. An X-ray machine can help diagnose and/or treat cancer.

Index